Official Journal of the

European Association of Urology

ESUR
European Society for Urological Research

EORTC
European Organization for Research and Treatment of Cancer – Genito-Urinary Group

European Urology

KARGER

Printed in Switzerland on acid-free paper by Reinhardt Druck, Basel

Appears monthly: 2 volumes per year (12 issues)

Guidelines for Authors

European Urology

Submission

Only original papers written in English are considered and should be sent to:

Prof. C.C. Schulman
S. Karger AG
Editorial Office European Urology
P.O. Box
CH–4009 Basel (Switzerland)
Tel. +41 61 306 1359
Fax +41 61 306 1434
E-Mail k.tschopp@karger.ch

Mailing address for courier deliveries only:

Allschwilerstr. 10
CH–4055 Basel (Switzerland)

Manuscripts should be submitted in triplicate (with three sets of illustrations of which one is an original), typewritten double-spaced on one side of the paper, with a wide margin.

Conditions

All manuscripts are subject to editorial review. Manuscripts are received with the explicit understanding that they are not under simultaneous consideration by any other publication. Submission of an article for publication implies the transfer of the copyright from the author to the publisher upon acceptance. Accepted papers become the permanent property of 'European Urology' and may not be reproduced by any means, in whole or in part, without the written consent of the publisher. It is the author's responsibility to obtain permission to reproduce illustrations, tables, etc. from other publications.

Original Papers: Should not exceed 3,500 words including tables and references.

Arrangement

Title page: The first page of each paper should indicate the title, the authors' names, and the institute where the work was conducted. A short title for use as running head as well as the full address of the author to whom correspondence should be sent are also required.

Full address: The exact postal address complete with postal code must be given at the bottom of the title page. Please also supply phone and fax numbers, as well as your e-mail address.

Key words: For indexing purposes, a list of 3–10 key words in English is essential.

Abstract: Each paper needs an abstract of up to 16 lines structured with subheadings as follows: Objective(s), Methods, Results, Conclusion(s).

Small type: Paragraphs which can or must be set in smaller type (case histories, test methods, etc.) should be indicated with a 'p' (petit) in the margin on the left-hand side.

Footnotes: Avoid footnotes. When essential, they are numbered consecutively and typed at the foot of the appropriate page.

Tables and illustrations: Tables and illustrations (both numbered in Arabic numerals) should be prepared on separate sheets. Tables require a heading and figures a legend, also prepared on a separate sheet. For the reproduction of illustrations, only good drawings and original photographs can be accepted; negatives or photocopies cannot be used. Due to technical reasons, figures with a screen background should not be submitted. When possible, group several illustrations on one block for reproduction (max. size 181 × 223 mm) or provide crop marks. On the back of each illustration, indicate its number, the author's name, and 'top' with a soft pencil.

Color illustrations: Up to 6 color illustrations per page can be integrated within the text at the reduced price of CHF 660.– / USD 545.00 per page. Color illustrations are reproduced at the author's expense.

References: In the text identify references by Arabic numerals [in square brackets]. Material submitted for publication but not yet accepted should be noted as 'unpublished data' and not be included in the reference list. The list of references should include only those publications which are cited in the text. Do not alphabetize; number references in the order in which they are first mentioned in the text. The surnames of the authors followed by initials should be given. There should be no punctuation other than a comma to separate the authors. Cite all authors, 'et al' is not sufficient. Abbreviate journal names according to the Index Medicus system. (Also see International Committee of Medical Journal Editors: Uniform requirements for manuscripts submitted to biomedical journals. N Engl J Med 1997;336:309–315.)

Examples
(a) Papers published in periodicals: Sun J, Koto H, Chung KF: Interaction of ozone and allergen challenges on bronchial responsiveness and inflammation in sensitised guinea pigs. Int Arch Allergy Immunol 1997;112:191–195.
(b) Monographs: Matthews DE, Farewell VT: Using and Understanding Medical Statistics, ed 3, revised. Basel, Karger, 1996.
(c) Edited books: Parren PWHI, Burton DR: Antibodies against HIV-1 from phage display libraries: Mapping of an immune response and progress towards antiviral immunotherapy; in Capra JD (ed): Antibody Engineering. Chem Immunol. Basel, Karger, 1997, vol 65, pp 18–56.

Rapid Communication: Manuscripts intended for rapid communication must present new findings of sufficient importance to justify their accelerated acceptance. They should follow the general arrangement of research papers. The first paragraph should include the reason for the study and the main findings. They should not exceed 8 double-spaced manuscript pages in length, including figures, tables and references. Review will be rapid, and once accepted, the paper will be included in the next planned issue.

Galley proofs

Unless otherwise indicated, galley proofs are sent to the first-named author and should be returned with the least possible delay. Alterations made in galley proofs, other than the correction of printer's errors, are charged to the author. No page proofs are supplied.

Reprints

Order forms and a price list are sent with the galley proofs. Orders submitted after the issue is printed are subject to considerably higher prices.

KARGER

Fax + 41 61 306 12 34
E-Mail karger@karger.ch
www.karger.com

The Guidelines for Authors are available at:
www.karger.com/journals/eur/eur_gl.htm

General Information

European
Urology

Publication data: 'European Urology' is published 12 times a year. Volumes 39–40 with 6 issues each appear in 2001.

Subscription rates: Subscriptions run for a full calendar year. Prices are given per volume.
Personal subscription:
Subscription + postage and handling
CHF 437.– + CHF 27.40 Europe
CHF 437.– + CHF 40.80 Overseas
USD 336.00 + USD 27.40
+ online subscription per volume:
CHF 39.– / USD 30.00
(Must be in the name of, billed to, and paid by an individual. Order must be marked 'personal subscription'.)
Institutional subscription:
Subscription + postage and handling
CHF 874.– + CHF 34.20 Europe
CHF 874.– + CHF 51.– Overseas
USD 672.00 + USD 34.20
+ online subscription per volume:
CHF 58.– / USD 45.00
Airmail postage: CHF 36.–, USD 30.00.
(Extra per volume.)
Discount subscription prices:
European Association of Urology
European Organization for Research and Treatment of Cancer – Genito-Urinary Group
European Society for Urological Research

Microforms: Please direct all enquiries and orders to: University Microfilms Inc.
300 North Zeeb Road, P.O. Box 1346
Ann Arbor, MI 48106-1346 (USA)

Subscription orders: Orders can be placed at agencies, bookstores, directly with the Publisher
S. Karger AG, P.O. Box,
CH–4009 Basel (Switzerland)
or with any of the following distributors:
Deutschland: S. Karger GmbH, Postfach
D–79095 Freiburg
France: Librairie Luginbühl
36, bd de Latour-Maubourg, F–75007 Paris
Great Britain, Ireland: S. Karger Publishers
58 Grove Hill Road
Tunbridge Wells, Kent TN1 1SP, UK
USA: S. Karger Publishers, Inc.
26 West Avon Road, P.O. Box 529
Farmington, CT 06085, USA
India, Bangladesh, Sri Lanka:
Panther Publishers Private Ltd.
39, 6th Cross
Wilson Gardens
Bangalore 560 027, India
Japan: Katakura Libri, Inc.
2F, Marushima Bldg, 4-6-17, Yushima,
Bunkyo-ku, Tokyo 113-0034, Japan

Change of address: Both old and new address should be sent to the subscription source.

Single issues and back volumes: Information can be obtained through the Publisher.

Advertising: Correspondence and rate requests should be addressed to the Publisher.

Bibliographic indices: This journal is regularly listed in bibliographic services, including *Current Contents®*.

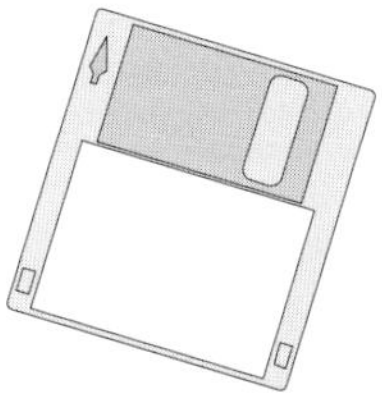

Disk Submission

A **comprehensive version** of these guidelines for the **submission of manuscripts and illustrations on disk** can be accessed online under **www.karger.com/journals/disksub.htm** or requested as a leaflet from the editorial department.

Please follow the general rules on style and arrangement in the **'Guidelines for Authors'** of the journal. Submit a **double-spaced printout** of your manuscript matching the file on disk exactly.

Technical Information
Store only data pertinent to this manuscript. Include your fonts (screen and printer fonts for Macintosh). For a **text only** manuscript, use a 3.5-inch disk. For **text and illustrations,** use 3.5 or 5.25 Magneto Optical Disc; CD-ROM (DOS or hybrid); iomage Zip/DOS (100 MB), or 44 MB, 88 MB or 200 MB SyQuest. Compress extensive data using ZIP format.

Data Description
Label your disk with the **title of the journal or book** for which it is submitted; a **short version** of the paper's title; your **name,** postal and e-mail address, fax and phone number; **hard and software** used, including the version; and the **complete list of the file names.** File names consist of eight characters before the dot identifying the file and three characters after the dot identifying the application.

Text and Format
The **preferred word-processing package is MS-Word.** Other commonly used PC text programs and ASCII formats are accepted.
Update your data when you revise subsequent to the reviewer's or editor's decision and mark revisions clearly. Manuscripts accepted for publication are subject to **copy editing:** changes and/or questions will be marked in the manuscript, which will be returned to you with your disk and the galley proofs for checking.
Enter your text continuously flush left. Do not use any layout functions. Do not split words at the end of a line. **Do not use indentations.** Use a blank line before and a hard return at the end of paragraphs. **Arrange headings flush left.** Insert only **one space after punctuation marks.** Insert Greek letters, mathematical symbols etc. with your word-processing program. Use **boldface and italics** as well as sub- and superscript where appropriate.
Tables are part of the text and should be placed at the end of the text file. Separate the individual parts of a table by lines. Use the tabulator instead of spaces. Format operation data on one line in the same column. **Legends to illustrations are part of the text** and should also be listed at the end of the text file.

Illustrations
Store illustrations as separate files: do not integrate them in your text. Export **line drawings/vector graphics** as TIF, EPS or WMF format. Use Photoshop for processing and retouching **scanned halftone images.** Save the original scan and the processed version. Export **black and white or color images** as TIF or EPS format in their anticipated size in print.
For detailed information on how to submit illustration data on disk please consult the leaflet or **www.karger.com/journals/disksub.htm.**

European
Urology

Triumph: Improving the Management of Lower Urinary Tract Symptoms in Real Life Practice

Guest Editor
C.R. Chapple, Sheffield

15 figures and 12 tables, 2001

KARGER

Basel · Freiburg · Paris · London · New York ·
New Delhi · Bangkok · Singapore · Tokyo · Sydney

Supported by an unconditional educational grant from Yamanouchi Europe B.V. and Boehringer Ingelheim International. Editorial support was provided by Ismar Healthcare N.V. The views and opinions expressed in this professional education supplement are those of the authors and do not necessarily reflect the views of Yamanouchi Europe B.V., Boehringer Ingelheim International or Ismar Healthcare.

S. Karger
Medical and Scientific Publishers
Basel · Freiburg · Paris · London
New York · New Delhi · Bangkok
Singapore · Tokyo · Sydney

Drug Dosage
The authors and the publisher have exerted every effort to ensure that drug selection and dosage set forth in this text are in accord with current recommendations and practice at the time of publication. However, in view of ongoing research, changes in government regulations, and the constant flow of information relating to drug therapy and drug reactions, the reader is urged to check the package insert for each drug for any change in indications and dosage and for added warnings and precautions. This is particularly important when the recommended agent is a new and/or infrequently employed drug.

P.O. Box, CH–4009 Basel (Switzerland)
Printed in Switzerland on acid-free paper by
Reinhardt Druck, Basel
ISBN 3–8055–7206–9

KARGER

Fax+ 41 61 306 12 34
E-Mail karger@karger.ch
www.karger.com

Vol. 39, Suppl. 3, 2001

European Urology

Contents

1 **Introduction and Conclusions**
Chapple, C.R. (Sheffield)

6 **Lower Urinary Tract Symptoms Suggestive of Benign Prostatic Obstruction: What Is the Available Evidence for Rational Management?**
Speakman, M.J. (Taunton)

13 **Lower Urinary Tract Symptoms Suggestive of Benign Prostatic Obstruction: How Can Clinical Expertise Contribute to Rational Management?**
Stoevelaar, H.J.; McDonnell, J.; Bosch, J.L.H.R. (Rotterdam); Kahan, J.P. (Leiden) and the European Panel on the Appropriate Treatment of BPH

20 **Lower Urinary Tract Symptoms Suggestive of Benign Prostatic Obstruction – What's the Long-Term Effectiveness of Medical Therapies?**
Michel, M.C.; Goepel, M. (Essen)

26 **Lower Urinary Tract Symptoms Suggestive of Benign Prostatic Obstruction: What Are the Current Practice Patterns?**
McNicholas, T.A. (Stevenage)

31 **Lower Urinary Tract Symptoms Suggestive of Benign Prostatic Obstruction – Triumph: Design and Implementation**
Chapple, C.R. (Sheffield) on behalf of the Pan-European Expert Panel

37 **Lower Urinary Tract Symptoms Suggestive of Benign Prostatic Obstruction – Triumph: Health-Economical Analysis**
McDonnell, J.; Busschbach, J.J.V.; Kok, E.; van Exel, J.; Stolk, E.; Koopmanschap, M.; Rutten, F.F.H. (Rotterdam)

42 **Lower Urinary Tract Symptoms Suggestive of Benign Prostatic Obstruction – Triumph: The Role of General Practice Databases**
Logie, J.W.; Clifford, G.M.; Farmer, R.D.T. (Guildford); Meesen, B.P.W. (Lier)

48 **Subject Index**

KARGER

Fax+41 61 306 12 34
E-Mail karger@karger.ch
www.karger.com

Access to full text and tables of contents, including tentative ones for forthcoming issues:
www.karger.com/journals/eur/eur_bk.htm

European Urology

Eur Urol 2001;39(suppl 3):1–5

Introduction and Conclusions

Christopher R. Chapple

Department of Urology, Royal Hallamshire Hospital, Sheffield, UK

Introduction

Symptomatic benign prostatic hyperplasia (BPH), nowadays often referred to as lower urinary tract symptoms (LUTS) suggestive of benign prostatic obstruction (BPO), is a very common condition in elderly men [1]. Due to the ageing of the population, the number of men suffering from LUTS will increase in the next millennium. Whilst about 15% of the population is currently aged 65 years or over, this proportion is expected to increase to 22% (range 19–25%) by 2025 [2]. In addition, these people will live longer and will expect a good quality of life (QoL) and appropriate medical care for the remainder of their (active) life. As a consequence the costs associated with the management of LUTS will increase substantially, whereas healthcare budgets will be relatively restricted. It will thus be a major challenge for the future to improve the cost-effective management of LUTS suggestive of BPO.

Currently, there are considerable differences between the management of LUTS suggestive of BPO across Europe in real life practice (RLP). For example, phytotherapy is particularly popular in France, Germany and Spain, while finasteride is often prescribed in Italy, Poland and the UK. Nevertheless, α_1-adrenoceptor antagonists are used in all these countries as a primary treatment modality [3]. These differences suggest that the current management of patients is very often more opinion- than evidence-based. A possible explanation for this might be that most evidence available today is based on classical efficacy (related to the effect on symptoms and urinary flow) and safety data of treatments coming from randomised controlled trials (RCTs) conducted on patients treated in secondary care, using protocols with strict inclusion/exclusion criteria. Consequently the study environment in RCTs does not reflect the patient population in RLP (fig. 1). The major drawback of RCTs is that results can not be readily generalised to clinical practice and as a consequence important questions at initiation of treatment in the real life patient population in primary care remain unanswered, which may at least partly explain the observed differences in prescribing/treatment behaviour seen across Europe. In the near future, more comparative

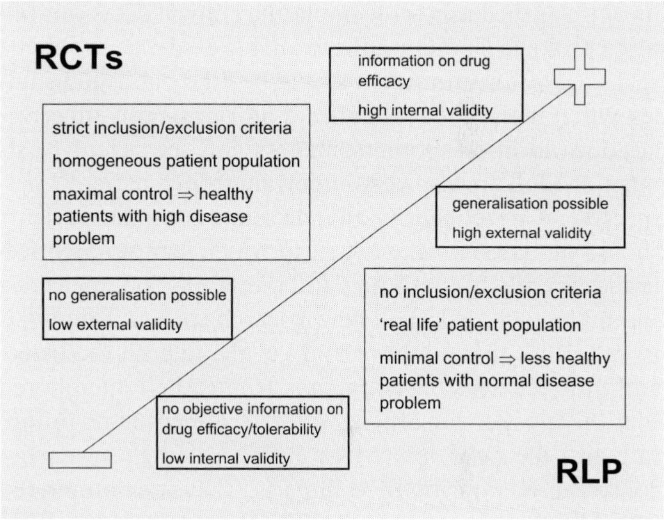

Fig. 1. Randomised controlled trials (RCTs) versus real life practice (RLP).

KARGER

Fax + 41 61 306 12 34
E-Mail karger@karger.ch
www.karger.com

0302–2838/01/0399–0001$17.50/0

Accessible online at:
www.karger.com/journals/eur

C.R. Chapple
Department of Urology, Royal Hallamshire Hospital
Glossop Road
Sheffield S10 2JF (UK)
Tel. +44 114 271 3047, Fax +44 114 279 7841, E-Mail c.r.chapple@sheffield.ac.uk

information is needed on the effectiveness of medical treatments in the long-term in order to allow us to develop specific hypotheses for evidence-based medicine (EBM) in RLP. It is well known that the effectiveness of treatment (i.e. reduction of complications related to BPO and switch to other medical therapy or surgery) is the major cost-driver in the management of LUTS suggestive of BPO.

Evidence-Based Medicine in LUTS

Bearing in mind the ageing of the population and the relatively restricted healthcare budgets, EBM will play a key role in improving cost-effective management of LUTS suggestive of BPO. EBM involves turning clinical problems into precise questions and then systematically locating, appraising and using contemporaneous research findings as the basis for formulating clinical decisions [4–6]. In urological practice, the available evidence should be reviewed by examining the strength of the published studies with reference to their efficacy and long-term effectiveness. In addition, bothersomeness and impact of treatment on QoL are also very important from a patient's perspective. Consequently, the decision to treat patients should be based on the extent to which symptoms interfere with daily life activities and therefore, QoL measures should be included in all new research studies. Finally, it is important that studies should evaluate both the direct and indirect costs of treatments. It must be remembered that the most costly aspect of any treatment is its failure rate and the need for re-treatment. Although an earlier consensus meeting on BPH in Paris [7] has recommended that all research papers on LUTS secondary to BPH should contain cost-effectiveness data, a review of the recent literature shows that this recommendation has not been implemented by most authors.

Based on the currently available evidence, transurethral resection of the prostate (TURP) remains the most effective treatment for de-obstructing patients, but the technique is less attractive from a patient's point of view [8]. Appropriate long-term data are still required to allow us to determine the ultimate position of most of the new, less invasive surgical techniques. Since medical therapy with either finasteride or α_1-adrenoceptor antagonists is not invasive as compared to surgery, this type of treatment is popular among patients. Both finasteride and α_1-adrenoceptor antagonists have a good efficacy and tolerability and are in the 'shorter' term more cost-efficient than TURP [9]. The use of finasteride has been suggested to be best restricted to patients with enlarged prostates (>40 ml) [10], while the efficacy of α_1-adrenoceptor antagonists is not dependent on prostate size [11–13]. Among the α_1-adrenoceptor antagonists, tamsulosin is now widely used and is the market leader as it has good tolerability and is safe with minimal cardiovascular effects and is easy to use (once daily administration without the need for stepwise dose increments on treatment initiation) [14, 15].

European Panel Study: Appropriateness of Therapy for LUTS

Widespread acceptance of EBM has been the stimulus for several organisations to develop practice guidelines, of which those of the AHCPR and the WHO are the most comprehensive and widely known [16, 17]. However, there still remains a large grey area of treatment choice in which no conclusive evidence exists on the right treatment for every patient. In this situation, the doctor's personal experiences, individual biases and training all act to complement evidence-based guidelines. By applying the RAND/UCLA method [18], the potential use of expert opinions in further guideline development for LUTS treatment has been assessed. The methodological background to this will be described in more detail by Stoevelaar et al. further on in this supplement [19]. Both a European panel and a Dutch panel rated the appropriateness of commonly available LUTS treatments for a large number of hypothetical patients. It appeared that both panels rated 84% of the indications identically. When no previous treatment was given, an α_1-adrenoceptor antagonist was considered to be the appropriate initial treatment in more than half of the cases. For cases in which α_1-adrenoceptor antagonist treatment failed, surgery was most frequently reported to be the appropriate therapy. Finasteride was considered inappropriate in a large number of cases, mainly in patients with small prostate volumes. It is encouraging that these observations are in accordance with the available evidence on the efficacy/tolerability ratio.

Long-Term Effectiveness of Treatments

Although LUTS suggestive of BPO progresses slowly, overall there is a slow background deterioration [20, 21]. Therefore in the management of LUTS it is not only important to consider the efficacy of treatment, but also the effectiveness of treatment in the longer-term. In particular, from a cost-effectiveness point of view it is very important to know how many patients develop complications due to BPO (e.g. AUR) or switch to other medical therapy or surgery. More information on these aspects is needed since these are the major cost-drivers in the management of LUTS suggestive of BPO [22].

The incidence of AUR during watchful waiting or in placebo arms of clinical trials is low, ranging between 0.5 and 3%/year, dependent on symptom severity and whether the study was community (0.7%/year) [23] or urologists' office based (1–2.5%/year) [24, 25]. Therefore, a large number of patients is needed to evaluate whether medical treatment can prevent the occurrence of AUR. Data from the PLESS study [26] demonstrate that finasteride treatment reduced the risk for AUR (from 7 to 3%) and surgery (from 10 to 5%). Whether α_1-adrenoceptor antagonists can also reduce the incidence of AUR or need for surgery has not been as intensively studied. One of the reasons for this might be that α_1-adrenoceptor antagonists, compared to finasteride, have a very fast onset of action (relief within 2–4 weeks) and consequently most trials with α_1-adrenoceptor antagonists have a relatively short follow-up (3–12 months). The direct comparative studies however indicate that α_1-adrenoceptor antagonists appear to have at least as positive an effect on disease progression as finasteride [11, 12]. A recently published 6-month study of 1,784 patients in an open study of tamsulosin demonstrated an incidence of AUR that was no higher than those values reported for finasteride [27].

The 'Medical Therapy of Prostatic Symptoms' (MTOPS) study, which is currently still ongoing, will hopefully allow us to retrieve more information on the impact of medical therapy on disease progression. This study should also be able to clarify whether long-term α-blockade results in the same risk reduction for AUR and surgery as finasteride. First results can be expected by the end of 2002 [28].

Triumph: Management of LUTS in RLP

The major shortage of available evidence today, both from an efficacy and effectiveness point of view, is due to the fact that all of these data are obtained in a secondary care setting and from RCTs. Therefore, the results are not easily generalisable to RLP where LUTS are managed by primary care physicians. In order to retrieve more information on cost-effectiveness of initial treatment modalities in real life primary care practice, the Triumph (Trans-european Research Into the Use of Management policies for LUTS suggestive of BPH in Primary Healthcare) project was established. This project will initially run in 6 European countries: France, Germany, Italy, Poland, Spain and the UK. The project has begun with an analysis of available general practice databases in France (THALES), The Netherlands (IPCI) and the UK (GPRD) to retrieve more information on both the incidence and prevalence of LUTS, its initial management and related long-term treatment failure. In addition, a prospective, cross-sectional, non-interventional survey will run in all 6 countries. Both newly diagnosed (n = 7,480) and existing patients, diagnosed with LUTS suggestive of BPO from January 1997 onwards (n = 5,480), will be prospectively followed for at least 1 year. Baseline characteristics (including I-PSS score), initial treatment choice and events related to disease progression will be collected. For the existing patients up to 3 years retrospective data concerning initial treatment, therapy switches and complications due to BPO will be retrieved from the patient medical records.

In order to assess the costs related to the management of LUTS, health-economists will develop a country-specific costing database for each of the participating countries [29]. These databases will contain estimates of the costs related to visits, investigations, medication, surgery, etc. This can be linked to data on patient characteristics and symptomatology at baseline and during follow-up to allow a cost-effectiveness analysis. In addition, a draft model will be developed based on the GPRD data that will enable, in combination with the national costing databases, country-specific health-economic analyses. This will be fine-tuned once the data from the observational survey become available. Finally, disease states will be developed and validated based on the I-PSS questionnaire that will enable quality adjusted life years (QALY's) calculation based on the I-PSS data collected in the prospective, observational survey. In a QALY-analysis, life years of a patient are 'corrected' for the value of quality of life, which usually varies from 0 (QoL equal to death) to 1 (QoL equal to normal health). In the Triumph project, QALYs are derived by converting health states of the I-PSS into QoL values based on the 'time trade-off' procedure. The validity of this method was initially tested on 100 male and female students. The students ranged the QoL-values from 0.83 for the worst LUTS-state to 0.96 for the best LUTS-state. Furthermore, the factor 'irritative' seemed to be rated as more severe than the factor 'obstructive', which is in line with literature data [30]. In a next step, the ratings of the general public were collected.

After completion of the analysis of these data, a final set of values specific for LUTS suggestive of BPO will be available, which can then be used in economic analyses within the Triumph project [29].

Triumph: Preliminary Results of the GPRD Study

Analysis of more than 60,000 older men included in the GPRD confirmed that the incidence and prevalence of LUTS increases with age. For the first time a linear relation was demonstrated. Furthermore, the incidence of prostatectomy also increased linearly from the age of 50 to 80 years, with a rate of 15 per 1,000 men at the age of 80. In the UK, the prescription of medical therapies has increased considerably over the last years and they are used earlier. This is probably a good tendency as the GPRD shows that patients receiving medical therapy have surgery at a later stage than patients initially receiving watchful waiting. Moreover, it appears that newer drugs, such as finasteride, alfuzosin and tamsulosin, are not only increasingly used, but are also associated with less treatment failure (i.e. less switch to other therapy, including surgery and less catheterisation) than older treatments such as indoramin and prazosin [31]. The prospective observational survey should act to confirm or refute these observations and will also give us insight into methodological biases such as possible confounding by indication, since in this study information on disease severity is collected at baseline through the I-PSS. Furthermore, for the first time this project will provide us with accurate data on real life practice, answering such questions as to how long individual patients stay on any particular therapy, which therapy, and how often they switch between therapies or progress on to surgery from medical therapy.

Conclusions

Due to the ageing and longevity of the population and the relatively restricted healthcare budgets, more rational management of LUTS suggestive of BPO is needed in the near future. In the framework of this, EBM is very important and should not only be based on efficacy and safety data from RCTs, but also on effectiveness of treatment as assessed in real life practice. Since there appears to be a shift in the initial management from secondary to primary care, more and better studies are needed in real life primary care practice. The Triumph project is one such attempt which will hopefully provide basic data and clinical directions which will enable us to improve the management of LUTS in the future.

References

1 Garraway WM, Collins GN, Lee RJ: High prevalence of benign prostatic hypertrophy in the community. Lancet 1991;338:469–471.

2 US Bureau of the Census (www.census.gov) (10/5/2000).

3 McNicholas T: LUTS suggestive of BPO. What are the current practice patterns? Eur Urol 2000;39(suppl 3):26–30.

4 Speakman MJ: LUTS suggestive of BPO. What is the available evidence for rational management? Eur Urol 2000;39(suppl 3):6–12.

5 Sackett DL, Rosenberg WM, Gray JA, Haynes RB, Richardson WS: Evidence based medicine: What it is and what it isn't. Br Med J 1996;312:71–72.

6 Rosenberg W, Donald A: Evidence based medicine: An approach to clinical problem solving. Br Med J 1995;310:1122–1126.

7 Cockett A, Khoury S, Aso Y, et al (eds): Proceedings of the 3th International Consultation on Benign Prostatic Hyperplasia (BPH): Monaco, 1995 Jun 26–28. Jersey Scientific Communication Ltd, 1996.

8 Bruskewitz R, Fourcade R, Koshiba K, Manyak M, Pisani E, Resel Estevez L, Vicente Rodriguez J: Surgery; in Denis L, Griffiths K, Khoury S, Cockett ATK, McConnell J, Chatelain C, Murphy G, Yoshida O (eds): Proceedings of the 4th International Consultation on Benign Prostatic Hyperplasia (BPH). Paris, 1997, Juli 2–5. Plymouth, Health Publication Ltd, 1998, pp 523–528.

9 Lowe FC, McDaniel RL, Chmiel JJ, Hillman AL: Economic modeling to assess the costs of treatment with finasteride, terazosin, and transurethral resection of the prostate for men with moderate to severe symptoms of benign prostatic hyperplasia. Urology 1995;46:477–483.

10 Boyle P, Gould AL, Roehrborn CG: Prostate volume predicts outcome of treatment of benign prostatic hyperplasia with finasteride: meta-analysis of randomized clinical trials. Urology 1996;48:398–405.

11 Lepor H, Williford WO, Barry MJ, Brawer MK, Dixon CM, Gormley G, Haakenson C, Machi M, Narayan P, Padley R: The efficacy of terazosin, finasteride or both in benign prostatic hyperplasia. N Engl J Med 1996:335:533–539.

12 Debruyne FMJ, Jardin A, Colloi D, Resel L, Witjes WPJ, Delauche-Cavallier MC, McCarthy C, Geffriaud-Ricouard C, on behalf of the European ALFIN Study Group: Sustained-release alfuzosin, finasteride and the combination of both in the treatment of benign prostatic hyperplasia. Eur Urol 1998;34:169–175.

13 Kirby R, Roehrborn C, Altwein JE, Bartsch G, Boyle P, Jardin A, for the PREDICT Investigators: Impact of prostate size on response to medical therapy for benign prostatic hyperplasia (BPH): Results of the PREDICT trial. J Urol 1999;161(suppl):266 (abstract 1028).

14 Djavan B, Marberger M: A meta-analysis on the efficacy and tolerability of α_1-adrenoceptor antagonists in patients with lower urinary tract symptoms suggestive of benign prostatic obstruction. Eur Urol 1999;36:1–13.

15 Lee M: Tamsulosin for the treatment of benign prostatic hypertrophy. Ann Pharmacother 2000;34:188–199.
16 McConnell JD, Barry MJ, Bruskewitz RC, et al. Clinical practice guideline for benign prostatic hyperplasia: Diagnosis and treatment. Rockeville, MD: Department of Health and Human Services, 1994. AHCPR publication No. 94–0582.
17 Cockett ATK, Aso Y, Chatelain C (eds): Proceedings of the 4th International Consultation on benign prostatic hyperplasia (BPH). Paris, 1997 Jul 2–5. Plumouth, Health Publication Ltd, 1998.
18 Kahn KL, Kosecoff J, Chassin MR, Flynn MF, Fink A, Pattaponghs N, Solomon DH, Brook RH: Measuring the clinical appropriateness of the use of a procedure. Can we do it? Med Care 1988;26:415–422.
19 Stoevelaar HJ, McDonnell J, Bosch JLHR, Kahan JP, and the European Panel on the Appropriate Treatment of BPH: LUTS suggestive of BPO. How can clinical expertise contribute to rational management? Eur Urol 2000;39(suppl 3):13–19.
20 Lee AJ, Garraway WM, Simpson RJ, Fisher W, King D: The natural history of untreated lower urinary tract symptoms in middle-aged and elderly men over a period of five years. Eur Urol 1998;34:325–332.
21 Jacobsen SJ, Girman CJ, Guess HA, Rhodes T, Oesterling JE, Lieber MM: Natural history of prostatism: Longitudinal changes in voiding symptoms in community dwelling men. J Urol 1996;155:595–600.
22 Michel MC, Goepel M: LUTS suggestive of BPO. What is the long-term effectiveness of medical therapies? Eur Urol 2000;39(suppl 3): 20–25.
23 Jacobsen SJ, Jacobsen DJ, Girman CJ, Roberts RO, Rhodes T, Guess HA, Lieber MM: Natural history of prostatism: Risk factors for acute urinary retention. J Urol 1997;158:481–487.
24 Barry MJ, Fowler FJ Jr, Bin L, Pitts JC III, Harris CJ, Mulley AG Jr: The natural history of patients with benign prostatic hyperplasia as diagnosed by North American urologists. J Urol 1997;157:10–15.
25 Wasson JH, Reda DJ, Bruskewitz RC, Elinson J, Keller AM, Henderson WG, for the Veterans Affairs Cooperative Study Group on transurethral resection of the prostate: A comparison of transurethral surgery with watchful waiting for moderate symptoms of benign prostatic hyperplasia. N Engl J Med 1995;332:75–79.
26 McConnell JD, Bruskewitz R, Walsh P, Andriole G, Lieber M, Holtgrewe L, Albertsen P, Roehrborn CG, Nickel JC, Wang DZ, Taylor AM, Waldstreicher J, for the PLESS Study Group: The effect of finasteride on the risk of acute urinary retention and the need for surgical treatment among men with benign prostatic hyperplasia. N Engl J Med 1998;338:557–563.
27 Michel MC, Bressel H-U, Goepel M, Rübben H: A 6-months large scale study into the safety of tamsulosin. Br J Clin Pharmacol 1999;48: 890P–891P.
28 MTOPS study: www.bsc.gwu.edu/mtops
29 McDonnell J, Busschbach JJV, Kok E, Exel J, Stolk E, Koopmanschap M, Rutten FFH: LUTS suggestive of BPO. Triumph: Health-economical analysis. Eur Urol 2000;39(suppl 3):37–41.
30 Reynard JM, Yang Q, Donovan JL, Peters TJ, Schafer W, de la Rosette JJMCH, Dabhoiwala NF, Osawa D, Tong Long Lim A, Abrams P: The ICS-BPH study: Uroflowmetry, lower urinary tract symptoms and bladder outlet obstruction. Br J Urol 1998;82:619–623.
31 Logie WJ, Clifford GM, Farmer RDT, Meesen BPW: LUTS suggestive of BPO. Triumph: The role of general practice databases. Eur Urol 2001;39(suppl 3):42–47.

European
Urology

Eur Urol 2001;39(suppl 3):6–12

Lower Urinary Tract Symptoms Suggestive of Benign Prostatic Obstruction: What Is the Available Evidence for Rational Management?

Mark J. Speakman

Taunton and Somerset Hospital, Taunton, UK

Key Words
LUTS · BPO · BPH · Evidence-based medicine · Rational management · Cost-effectiveness

Abstract
Because of the need for a more rational management of LUTS suggestive of BPO, EBM is receiving more attention. Treatment decisions should be based on scientific evidence more than on personal preferences of physicians and patients. EBM is more than following rigid treatment guidelines or published advice. It is a process of turning problems of clinical practice into well-defined questions and then finding and appraising available evidence and implementing it into clinical practice. In cases of LUTS suggestive of BPO, much evidence is available on the efficacy and tolerability of different treatment modalities in the short term, whereas long-term data on (cost)-effectiveness are rather scarce. From a patient's point of view, newer pharmacotherapeutic agents can be considered as an appropriate treatment option. α_1-Adrenoceptor antagonists seem to be more efficacious than finasteride and within this group of drugs, selective α_{1A}/α_{1D}-adrenoceptor antagonists particularly show a favourable efficacy/tolerability ratio.

Introduction

The management of lower urinary tract symptoms (LUTS) suggestive of benign prostatic obstruction (BPO), a highly prevalent condition in older men [1], is nowadays an important cost driver in healthcare budgets and because the population is ageing, it will claim even more of the budget in the next millennium. Currently, LUTS suggestive of BPO, previously also referred to as benign prostatic hyperplasia (BPH), can be managed by various therapies, including invasive (e.g. open surgery, transurethral resection of the prostate (TURP)) and minimally invasive therapies (e.g. laser therapy, thermotherapy), medical treatments (5α-reductase inhibitors, α_1-adrenoceptor antagonists, phytotherapy) or watchful waiting (close follow-up of the patient without active treatment). Consequently, physicians and patients have a wide range of choices to manage LUTS, each with a different cost pattern. Nowadays, the choice of therapy for a certain patient still seems to depend a great deal on personal and cultural preferences of the physician and the patient. Phytotherapy for example is regularly used in France, Germany and Spain where it is registered and reimbursed, whereas it is less frequently used in Italy and Poland and not prescribed at all in the UK. Finasteride is more commonly used in Italy, the UK and Poland than in France, Germany and Spain, where its market share is rather small. The only similarity

KARGER

Fax + 41 61 306 12 34
E-Mail karger@karger.ch
www.karger.com

0302–2838/01/0399–0006$17.50/0

Accessible online at:
www.karger.com/journals/eur

M.J. Speakman
Taunton and Somerset Hospital
Musgrove Park
Taunton, Somerset TA1 5DA (UK)
Tel. +44 1823 342102, Fax +44 1823 343571, E-Mail speakmanmj@aol.com

in prescription patterns between those six countries (and other European countries) is the high market share of α_1-adrenoceptor antagonists [2]. In addition, the incidence of surgery has declined world-wide since the penetration on the world market of improved pharmacotherapies [3].

The population in the industrialised world is ageing: in Western Europe for example, the percentage of men ≥65 years represents 13.5% of the total male population in 2000 whereas this is estimated to increase up to 20.2% in 2025 [4]. In addition, fewer younger working people will have to take care of a larger number of older people. Consequently, healthcare budgets will be relatively restricted in the future and a more cost-effective healthcare delivery will thus be required. This is especially valid for the management of LUTS suggestive of BPO as the number of elderly men presenting, suffering from LUTS is growing enormously. There is also a demand for the highest quality of treatment and care. As a result, evidence-based medicine (EBM) is now receiving more attention in the field of LUTS suggestive of BPO.

This paper tries to outline some general issues about EBM as well as the current status of EBM in the management of LUTS suggestive of BPO. Which information is already available and what is still largely lacking?

Evidence-Based Medicine

Definition

To improve the quality and (cost)-efficiency of healthcare delivery, physicians and healthcare planners need to use more and more available research evidence as a tool for clinical decision making. In this perspective, EBM aims to integrate current best evidence from research with clinical expertise, pathophysiological knowledge and patient preferences in making decisions about the care of individual patients and within general healthcare policy [5, 6]. As such, EBM should be derived from a combination of available external clinical evidence obtained from scientific literature on the one hand and individual clinical experience of similar patient situations on the other hand. Also very important is the fact that EBM involves patient participation in health decision-making at all levels [7]. Thus, medicine based on scientific evidence is much more complicated than just following broad guidelines, such as the valuable guidelines from the AHRQ (Agency for Healthcare Research and Quality, formerly AHCPR or Agency for Health Care Policy and Research) or following the advice from the latest publication in a major journal. David Sackett and colleagues [8] defined EBM as '... the conscientious, explicit and judicious use of current best evidence in making decisions about the care of individual patients'.

Process of EBM

The process of finding, assessing, interpreting and applying current best evidence in clinical practice is not an easy one. In general, the process of EBM involves several steps to be taken by the physician or healthcare planner. First, the information needs have to be converted into accurate questions, in order to perform a thorough and complete literature search to come eventually to correct conclusions. Secondly, the best evidence has to be tracked down from the most appropriate source (e.g. MEDLINE®, Cochrane) efficiently using the available information technology. Third, one must critically appraise the evidence for its validity (i.e. closeness to the truth) and its usefulness (i.e. clinical applicability) and fourth, the results of this appraisal must be integrated with clinical expertise and applied in clinical practice. Finally, an evaluation of the performance is necessary.

Evidence Gathering

Much evidence is available nowadays, but unfortunately not everything is of high scientific value and/or can pass the test of 'clinical relevance'. Many studies are not properly designed and are not performed according to good clinical practice (GCP) guidelines, which makes their scientific value doubtful. As such, it can be difficult, though it is a very important task for physicians and healthcare decision makers to search and select that evidence that is valuable for his/her problem. To gather such relevant evidence, it is obvious that computer media and the Internet are nowadays indispensable. Many commercial CD-ROM databases and Internet database subscriptions with world-wide information are available at present, such as the EMBASE® database which is a comprehensive index of the world's literature on human medicine and related disciplines and can be consulted via The Dialog Corporation [http://www.dialog.com]. On some websites however, very useful evidence of high scientific value can be found without the need for subscription. For example, the abstracts and references in the MEDLINE® database, i.e, the U.S. National Library of Medicine's (NLM) bibliographic database that contains over 11 million references to journal articles in life sciences with emphasis on biomedicine, can be consulted for free via PubMed [http://www.ncbi.nlm.nih.gov/entrez/query.fcgi]. Also the websites of the AHRQ, formerly known as the AHCPR [http://www.ahcpr.gov] and the Cochrane library

Table 1. Strength of evidence in EBM

I	Strong evidence – at least 1 systematic review of RCTs
II	Strong evidence – at least 1 RCT
III	Evidence from non-randomised trials, cohort studies, time series or case-controlled studies
IV	Evidence from non-experimental studies
V	Opinion-audit, descriptive studies or expert committees

(see below) [http://www.cochrane.org/cochrane/cdsr.htm] are valuable sources of relevant healthcare information.

Ranking Evidence

The evidence used in EBM has been subdivided into five stages of scientific value or credibility (see table 1). The best evidence (level I) comes from systematic reviews or meta-analyses of well-designed randomised controlled trials (RCTs) comparing the active treatment with placebo and/or an alternative available treatment. The second level (level II) consists of individual properly designed RCTs, which are still considered as the 'gold standard' to obtain scientific evidence for initial evaluation of a new therapy in order to define its efficacy/safety ratio. RCTs have strict inclusion and exclusion criteria and hence are a perfect tool for assessing the impact of the investigated treatment(s) on the dependent variables with or without minimal influence of external factors. They are perfect in assessing the efficacy of a treatment. On the other hand, we must not forget that RCTs are in general performed in small homogeneous patient groups that are most of the time not a realistic reflection of the real life patient situation in clinical practice. Many of the patients ultimately treated would have been excluded from RCTs because of multiple co-morbidities or co-medications. The fact that rather small patient groups are used makes it also impossible to detect side effects that occur in few patients and to perform meaningful subgroup analyses, such as tolerability in elderly or in patients with cardiovascular co-morbidity and/or co-medication. Therefore, data obtained from large-scale studies performed in real life practice (RLP) can also add considerable extra value to the available evidence from RCTs. Such evidence is situated at the evidence levels III and IV, standing respectively for evidence from cohort studies or case-controlled studies and evidence from non-experimental studies. Next to RCTs, we need information from these studies to confirm the efficacy and probably even more important safety and long-term effectiveness of the treatment in clinical practice. Finally, data from opinion-audits, descriptive studies or expert committees represent the level V of evidence and may represent 'standard' practice of selected physicians. If however, expert committees draw up guidelines from level I advice from systematic reviews, then their validity may rise up towards level I evidence. In decision-making costs also play an increasingly important role.

This attempt to rank evidence in different levels should however be interpreted very carefully. Bias can creep into reviews or meta-analyses. For example, negative results are still relatively rarely published and are thus largely omitted from these publications. There also often seems to be language bias where papers written in languages other than English may carry less weight in a meta-analysis.

The Cochrane Collaboration

As mentioned before, reviews of well-designed RCTs are nowadays considered as the best source of initial evidence. As such, the Cochrane Library, which contains regularly updated systematic reviews of the effects of healthcare, can be considered as a valuable source of information.

Archie Cochrane, a British epidemiologist and founder of the Cochrane Collaboration, recognised that there was a lot of information available from different RCTs, but that the information should be brought together in reviews in order to be fully useful for healthcare decisions. In 1979 he wrote [9]: 'It is surely a great criticism of our profession that we have not organised a critical summary, by speciality or subspecialty, adapted periodically, of all relevant randomised controlled trials.' He referred to a systematic review of RCTs on care during pregnancy and childbirth as 'a real milestone in the history of randomised trials and in the evaluation of care.' He also suggested that other fields of medicine should put emphasis on reviews of research evidence that must be prepared systematically and should be kept up-to-date with the latest research information. The Cochrane Collaboration [10] addresses this need for internationally organised healthcare information and has developed a call for systematic up-to-date reviews of all relevant RCTs. As such, this international organisation aims to help people make well informed decisions about healthcare by preparing, maintaining and ensuring the accessibility of systematic reviews. All over the world, over 40 Collaborative Cochrane Review Groups, covering most of the important areas of healthcare, prepare and maintain the Cochrane reviews. These groups consist of researchers, healthcare professionals, consumers and others, all willing to provide reliable and up-to-date evidence in the prevention, treatment and rehabilitation of health problems. All the full Cochrane reviews are kept in the electronic Cochrane Library, which is published quarterly on CD-ROM or on the Internet and which can be consulted after subscription. The abstracts of the reviews are accessible for free for every Internet user (for example, on the Cochrane library website or the MEDLINE® database; see above). Each review/protocol incorporated into the Cochrane Database of Systematic Reviews has a standardised structure.

One of the Cochrane Collaborative Review Groups is the Cochrane Prostatic and Urologic Cancers Group, coordinated by R. MacDonald (Department of Veterans' Affairs Medical Center, Minneapolis, USA). This group has already prepared several reviews and protocols (i.e. the introduction, objectives, materials and methods for reviews that are in preparation) concerning research evidence from RCTs on treatments for different urologic and prostatic diseases. As illustration, table 2 gives the available reviews and protocols in the field of LUTS suggestive of BPO.

Table 2. Cochrane reviews and protocols in the field of LUTS suggestive of BPO

Reviews
Beta-sitosterols for benign prostatic hyperplasia
Cernilton for benign prostatic hyperplasia
Serenoa repens for benign prostatic hyperplasia
Protocols
Laser prostatectomy for benign prostatic hyperplasia*
Pygeum africanum for benign prostatic hyperplasia
Tamsulosin for benign prostatic hyperplasia#
Terazosin for benign prostatic hyperplasia

* Review will be released the 4th quarter of 2000.
\# Review will be released the 1st quarter of 2001.

EBM in the Management of LUTS Suggestive of BPO

Active Treatment versus Watchful Waiting

For individual patients with LUTS suggestive of BPO different management approaches can and should be considered. A treatment strategy that is appropriate for one patient might be completely irrelevant for another. As such, the physician together with the patient should first analyse whether the patient really needs an active treatment or if he can better be followed closely without undergoing surgery or receiving medication, i.e. a watchful waiting strategy. The progression of symptoms and obstruction is not universal and some patients might even improve over time without receiving any therapy [11, 12]. Thus, reassurance and a watchful waiting strategy may be a reasonable option. Important criteria when selecting whether or not a patient may benefit from an active treatment are symptom severity, preferably assessed via the International Prostate Symptom Score (I-PSS) [13], the actual bother for the patient, assessed via the Symptom Problem Index (SPI) [14] and/or the patient's quality of life (QoL) or the impact on daily life activities, assessed through the I-PSS-QoL question [15] or the BPH Impact Index (BPI) [14]. These factors should be balanced against treatment morbidity or possible side effects. For example, a patient with a high symptom score and a significant bother factor will accept considerably more morbidity after a surgical procedure or complain much less about some minor adverse events of a drug therapy than a patient with minimal symptoms and bother.

Treatment Outcomes

In order to review different treatments for LUTS suggestive of BPO, valuable data from published studies are required concerning the efficacy and tolerability of treatment options (i.e. the effect on both subjective symptoms and urinary flow and the incidence of adverse effects), the long-term effectiveness, the impact on daily life activities (QoL) and the costs. The efficacy and tolerability of invasive or medical therapies are predominantly obtained from large-scale RCTs in a secondary care setting which have a high internal validity or reproducibility. Although very important and indispensable to estimate the initial value of a treatment, this evidence is not sufficient in a real life clinical practice. Also long-term results should be evaluated, with special emphasis on the failure rate of treatments, assessed through the switch to other medical therapy or surgery and/or the delay or prevention of complications related to BPO such as acute urinary retention (AUR). It has been assumed that a cascade of treatments is the most costly management option for LUTS suggestive of BPO, which indicates that, from a cost-effectiveness point of view, this should be avoided wherever possible. In addition, QoL measures are essential as they estimate the actual bother and improvement of bother for the patient. A therapy that for example improves the urinary flow of the patient but does not improve his QoL may be considered as a waste of money. Finally, evidence concerning the direct and indirect costs of treatment options is needed as well as the intangible costs on the patients

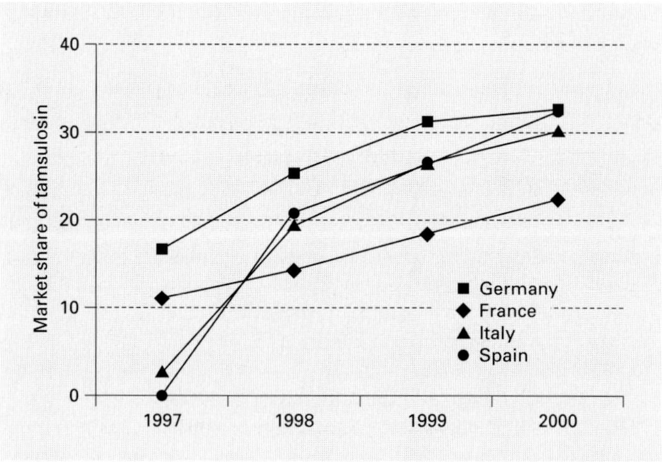

Fig. 1. Market share of tamsulosin in some European countries.

and their families. Especially in the light of the increasing prevalence of LUTS suggestive of BPO and relatively restricted healthcare budgets in the future, this is a very important issue. Although an earlier consensus meeting on BPH in Paris has recommended that papers on LUTS suggestive of BPO should contain cost-effectiveness data [3], this recommendation has hardly been taken up so far.

Available/Missing Evidence

At present, much information is available on the (short-term) efficacy and tolerability of different therapies whereas QoL measures and information concerning the long-term effectiveness are largely lacking for most therapies. Also analyses on the cost-effectiveness, i.e. the balance of the gain and the costs of a treatment, are rather scarce.

Based on the available evidence today, transurethral resection of the prostate (TURP) is still considered as 'the gold standard' and very effective in relieving symptoms and improving urinary flow in patients with LUTS suggestive of BPO [16]. However, many patients are not very keen on undergoing an operation and possible negative and bothersome side effects such as incontinence or impotence should be taken into consideration when choosing this option [17]. More recently, newer and so-called less invasive surgical techniques have been developed and introduced. These techniques appear to be less effective than TURP and require more re-treatments, but on the other hand other aspects such as a reduced risk of blood transfusion, the need for only local anaesthesia or a shorter hospital stay should be balanced against this reduction in efficacy. To appraise the ultimate position of these techniques in LUTS management, more unbiased and properly designed short-term and particularly long-term 'sham'-controlled, large clinical studies are needed. During the last decade, more and more attention has been given to the medical treatment of LUTS suggestive of BPO and a lot is published on pharmacotherapy. For example, more than 180 papers were published and catalogued in MEDLINE® during the last ten years (1990–2000) on tamsulosin, the latest developed medical agent and the first subtype selective α_{1A}/α_{1D}-adrenoceptor antagonist for the treatment of LUTS suggestive of BPO. Based on the contemporary available evidence, both finasteride and α_1-adrenoceptor antagonists (respectively 700+ and 500+ papers in MEDLINE®) are effective, reasonably well tolerated and in the 'shorter' term more cost-effective than TURP [11, 18]. Evidence regarding the cost-effectiveness in the 'longer' term is however lacking. Comparing these two medical therapies, the available evidence suggests that α_1-adrenoceptor antagonists are more effective than finasteride, irrespective of prostate size, while the use of finasteride should be limited to patients with enlarged prostates (>40 ml) [19–22]. The effects of treatments on the prevention of AUR or the need for surgery are discussed in detail in the paper of M.C. Michel and M. Goepel, published in this supplement [23]. In addition, α_1-adrenoceptor antagonists have a very fast onset of action. In the case of tamsulosin, in addition to papers on efficacy and tolerability in RCTs, specific effects of the drug were also examined and published, such as effects on blood pressure regulation and ambulatory stress testing, effects on sexual function and QoL, effects in diabetic patients, patients with cardiovascular comorbidity and/or comedication and in the elderly [24–30]. These data indicate that a single daily dose of 0.4 mg tamsulosin (without dose titration) has a good efficacy, equivalent to other, non-subtype selective α_1-adrenoceptor antagonists, but seems to have a more favourable side effect profile, including in special patient groups. Also the market is valuing these positive results for tamsulosin, as the market share of the drug is currently growing in Germany, France, Italy and Spain (see fig. 1) [2]. Here also however, valuable information on the (cost)-effectiveness of tamsulosin as initial treatment modality is still missing. Finally, only a few properly designed placebo-controlled trials with plant extracts have been performed and long-term trials are (still) lacking. The Cochrane Review on Cernilton, prepared from the rye-grass pollen *Secale cereale,* asserts that reliable evidence is missing because the trials analysed are not well designed [31]. Evidence from clinical trials of *Serenoa repens* suggests an improvement of the urinary flow rate compared to placebo, but insufficient data are available concerning symptom score improvement and the long-term effectiveness, safety and ability to prevent complications related to BPO [32, 33]. Also substantial short/long-term data retrieved from adequately performed RCTs with β-sitosterol are rather scarce [34, 35].

Conclusion

The concept of EBM dictates that clinical decisions are based more on scientific research evidence than on tradition and personal preferences. On this point of view, the guidelines of the WHO International Consultations and the AHRQ (formerly known as the AHCPR) are a valuable source of information to help healthcare decision-makers in their choices. In case of LUTS suggestive of BPO, already a lot of evidence on the efficacy and tolerability of different treatment options is available particularly in the short-term while long-term data and cost-effectiveness data of treatments are still largely lacking. According to the available evidence, α_1-adrenoceptor antagonists are an attractive therapeutic option from a patient's point of view and especially the newer drugs such as tamsulosin and alfuzosin show a favourable efficacy/tolerability ratio and are very convenient in use (once daily administration and no dose titration). The insufficiency of long-term research evidence may be seen as a considerable limitation of EBM and treatment guidelines today. In addition, many patients belong to a 'grey area' of the population of men with LUTS, for which it is impossible to follow guidelines on how they should be best treated. To fill these gaps, a complementation of clinical research evidence and treatment guidelines by the personal experiences and insights of physicians is desirable. A perfect tool for that may be the analysis of panel studies regarding the appropriateness of therapy for LUTS suggestive of BPO, as discussed in the paper of H.J. Stoevelaar in this supplement [36]. In conclusion, the combination of scientific research evidence and clinical experience may be the cornerstone for good EBM and rational clinical management.

References

1 Garraway WM, Collins GN, Lee RJ: High prevalence of benign prostatic hypertrophy in the community. Lancet 1991;338:469–471.
2 IMS/GERS market analysis data, March 2000.
3 Holtgrewe HL, Bay-Nielsen H, Carlsson P, Coast J, Echtle D, Fitzpatrick F, Lanson Y, Melchior H, Standaert B, Vallancien G: The economics of the management of lower urinary tract symptoms and benign prostatic hyperplasia; in Denis L, Griffiths K, Khoury S, Cockett ATK, McConnell J, Chatelain C, Murphy G, Yoshida O (eds): Proceedings of the 4th International Consultation on BPH. Plymouth, Plymbridge Distributors Ltd, 1998, pp 63–81.
4 U.S. Bureau of the Census, International Data Base (August 2000): http://www.census.gov.
5 Ellrodt G, Cook DJ, Lee J, Cho M, Hunt D, Weingarten S: Evidence-based disease management. JAMA 1997;278:1687–1692.
6 Haynes B, Haines A: Getting research findings into practice. Barriers and bridges to evidence based clinical practice. BMJ 1998;317:273–276.
7 Hirst GHL, Ward, JE: Clinical practice guidelines: Reality bites. Med J Aust 2000;172:287–291.
8 Sackett DL, Rosenberg WM, Gray JA, Haynes RB, Richardson WS: Evidence based medicine: What it is and what it isn't. BMJ 1996; 312(7023):71–72.
9 Cochrane AL: 1931–1971: A critical review, with particular reference to the medical profession; in Medicines for the year 2000. London, Office of Health Economics, 1979, pp 1–11.
10 http://www.cochrane.org.
11 Speakman MJ: Who should be treated and how? Evidence-based medicine in symptomatic BPH. Eur Urol 1999;36(suppl 3):40–51.
12 Barry MJ, Fowler FJ, Bin L, Pitts JC, Harris CJ, Mulley AG: The natural history of patients with benign prostatic hyperplasia as diagnosed by North American urologists. J Urol 1997; 157:10–15.
13 Denis L, McConnell J, Yoshida O, Khoury S, Abrams P, Barry M, Bartsch G, Cockett A, Corriere J, Dreikorn K, Gibbons R, Griffiths K, Hald T, Holtgrewe L, Jardin A, Koyanagi T, Mebust W, Murphy G, Roehrborn C, Smyth P, The Members of the Committees. Recommendations of the International Scientific Committee: The evaluation and treatment of lower urinary tract symptoms (LUTS) suggestive of benign prostatic obstruction; in Denis L, Griffiths K, Khoury S, Cockett ATK, McConnell J, Chatelain C, Murphy G, Yoshida O (eds): Proceedings of the 4th International Consultation on BPH. Plymouth, Plymbridge Distributors Ltd, 1998, pp 669–684.
14 Barry MJ, Fowler FJ, O'Leary MP, Bruskewitz RC, Holtgrewe HL, Mebust WK: Measuring disease-specific health status in men with benign prostatic hyperplasia. Med Care 1995;33: AS145–155.
15 Barry MJ, Fowler FJ, O'Leary MP, Bruskewitz RC, Holtgrewe HL, Mebust WK, Cockett AT: The American Urological Association symptom index for benign prostatic hyperplasia. J Urol 1992;148:1549–1557.
16 Djavan B, Madersbacher S, Klingler HC, Ghawidel K, Basharkhah A, Hruby S, Seitz C, Marberger M: Outcome analysis of minimally invasive treatments for benign prostatic hyperplasia. Tech Urol 1999;5:12–20.
17 Chapple CR: Medical therapy and quality of life. Eur Urol 1998;34(suppl 2):10–17.
18 Lowe FC, McDaniel RL, Chmiel JJ, Hillman AL: Economic modeling to assess the costs of treatment with finasteride, terazosin, and transurethral resection of the prostate for men with moderate to severe symptoms of benign prostatic hyperplasia. Urology 1995;46:477–483.
19 Lepor H, Williford WO, Barry MJ, Brawer MK, Dixon CM, Gormley G, Haakenson C, Machi M, Narayan P, Padley R: The efficacy of terazosin, finasteride or both in benign prostatic hyperplasia. N Engl J Med 1996:335:533–539.
20 Debruyne FMJ, Jardin A, Colloi D, Resel L, Witjes WPJ, Delauche-Cavallier MC, McCarthy C, Geffriaud-Ricouard C, on behalf of the European ALFIN Study Group: Sustained-release alfuzosin, finasteride and the combination of both in the treatment of benign prostatic hyperplasia. Eur Urol 1998;34:169–175.

21 Kirby R, Jens EA, Bartsch G, Boyle P, Jardin A, Roehrborn C, for the PREDICT Investigators: Results of the PREDICT (Prospective European doxazosin and combination therapy) trial. J Urol 1999;16(suppl 4):266 (abstract 1027).
22 Boyle P, Gould AL, Roehrborn CG: Prostate volume predicts outcome of treatment of benign prostatic hyperplasia with finasteride: Meta-analysis of randomized clinical trials. Urology 1996;48:398–405.
23 Michel MC, Goepel M: Lower urinary tract symptoms suggestive of benign prostatic obstruction – What's the long-term effectiveness of medical therapies? Eur Urol 2001;39(suppl 3):20–25.
24 Djavan B, Marberger M: A meta-analysis on the efficacy and tolerability of α_1-adrenoceptor antagonists in patients with lower urinary tract symptoms suggestive of benign prostatic obstruction. Eur Urol 1999;36:1–13.
25 Höfner K, Claes H, De Reijke TM, Folkestad B, Speakman MJ: Tamsulosin 0.4 mg once daily: Effect on sexual function in patients with lower urinary tract symptoms suggestive of benign prostatic obstruction. Eur Urol 1999;36: 335–341.
26 Michel MC, Mehlburger L, Schumacher H, Bressel HU, Goepel M: Effect of diabetes on lower urinary tract symptoms in patients with benign prostatic hyperplasia. J Urol 2000;163: 1725–1729.
27 Michel MC, Mehlburger L, Bressel H-U, Schumacher H, Schäfers RF, Goepel M: Tamsulosin treatment of 19,365 patients with lower urinary tract symptoms: does co-morbidity alter tolerability? J Urol 1998;160:784–791.
28 Michel MC, Bressel H-U, Mehlburger L, Goepel M: Tamsulosin: Real life clinical experience in 19,365 patients. Eur Urol 1998;34(suppl 2): 37–45.
29 Lowe FC: Coadministration of tamsulosin and three antihypertensive agents in patients with benign prostatic hyperplasia: Pharmacodynamic effect. Clin Ther 1997;19:730–742.
30 Chapple CR, Baert L, Thind P, Höfner K, Khoe GSS, Spangberg A: Tamsulosin 0.4 mg once daily: Tolerability in older and younger patients with lower urinary tract symptoms suggestive of benign prostatic obstruction (symptomatic BPH). Eur Urol 1997;32:462–470.
31 Wilt T, MacDonald R, Ishani A, Rutks I, Stark G: Cernilton for benign prostatic hyperplasia (Cochrane Review). Cochrane Database Syst Rev 2000,3.
32 Boyle P, Robertson C, Lowe, F, Roehrborn: Meta-analysis of clinical trials of Permixon in the treatment of symptomatic benign prostatic hyperplasia. Urology 2000;55:533–539.
33 Wilt T, Ishani A, Stark G, MacDonald R, Mulrow C, Lau J: Serenoa repens for benign prostatic hyperplasia (Cochrane Review). Cochrane Database Syst Rev 2000,3.
34 Wilt T, Ishani A, MacDonald R, Stark G, Mulrow C, Lau J: β-Sitosterols for benign prostatic hyperplasia (Cochrane Review). Cochrane Database Syst Rev 2000,3.
35 Wilt T, MacDonald R, Ishani A: β-sitosterol for the treatment of benign prostatic hyperplasia: A systematic review. BJU Int 1999;83:976–983.
36 Stoevelaar HJ, McDonnell J, Bosch JLHR, Kahan JP: Lower urinary tract symptoms suggestive of benign prostatic obstruction: How can experience contribute to rational management? Eur Urol 2001;39(suppl 3):13–19.

European Urology

Eur Urol 2001;39(suppl 3):13–19

Lower Urinary Tract Symptoms Suggestive of Benign Prostatic Obstruction: How Can Clinical Expertise Contribute to Rational Management?

H.J. Stoevelaar[a] J. McDonnell[a] J.L.H.R. Bosch[b] J.P. Kahan[c]
and the European Panel on the Appropriate Treatment of BPH[1]

[a]Institute for Health Care Policy and Management, Erasmus University, Rotterdam, [b]Department of Urology, University Hospital Rotterdam, Rotterdam, and [c]RAND Europe, Leiden, The Netherlands

Key Words
Benign prostatic hyperplasia · Practice guidelines · Clinical decision making · LUTS

Abstract
Objective: To perform a systematic analysis of clinical expertise on treatment for benign prostatic hyperplasia (lower urinary tract symptoms (LUTS) suggestive of benign prostatic obstruction (BPO)) and to investigate the usefulness of these data in further guideline development. ***Methods:*** A modified Delphi method was used to analyse the opinions of a panel of 15 European urologists on the appropriateness of 4 common treatments for 1,152 'indications' (hypothetical cases) for LUTS suggestive of BPO. Each indication consisted of a unique combination of 9 diagnostic variables, found to be relevant in treatment choice in previous research. The study population was restricted to patients for whom current guidelines do not provide clear indications on the most appropriate treatment. The panellists individually rated the appropriateness of three active treatments (surgery, α_1-adrenoceptor antagonists, finasteride) using a 9-point scale, all in comparison with 'watchful waiting'. Aggregate panel judgements were calculated from individual ratings for each indication (appropriate, inappropriate, and uncertain). The relationship between diagnostic characteristics and panel opinions was analysed using logistic regression methods. The results were compared to those of an identical panel study including 12 Dutch urologists. ***Results:*** Strong agreement existed for 42.5% of the indications, while strong disagreement was found in only 0.1%. For patients who had not previously been treated for LUTS, surgery was considered appropriate in 44% of the indications. For α_1-adrenoceptor antagonists and finasteride these percentages were 56 and 6 respectively. Strong contra-indications were found only for finasteride (34%). Logistic regression analysis demonstrated consistent panel opinions, indicating a strong cumulative impact of almost all diagnostic variables on the panel judgement 'appropriate'. The figures on appropriateness were highly comparable to the results of the Dutch study (overall agreement 84%, kappa 0,76). A computer program was constructed to facilitate the implementation and evaluation of the panel recommendations in daily clinical practice. ***Conclusions:*** Given the consistency of the panel opinions, the results may be

[1] *European Panel on the Appropriate Treatment of BPH:* J.E. Batista (Barcelona, Spain), T. Berggren (Halmstad, Sweden), J.H.M. Blom (Rotterdam, The Netherlands), W. du Fossé (Leiden, The Netherlands), P. de Geeter (Kassel, Germany), F.C. Hamdy (Sheffield, United Kingdom), N. Harrison (Lewes, United Kingdom), M.T.W.T. Lock (Utrecht, The Netherlands), T.A. McNicholas (Hitchin, United Kingdom), J. Moreno Sierra (Madrid, Spain), R. Muschter (Rotenberg, Germany), L. Rentzhog (Sundsvall, Sweden), J. Salinas (Madrid, Spain), P.J.R. Shah (London, United Kingdom), A. Spangberg (Linköping, Sweden).

KARGER
Fax + 41 61 306 12 34
E-Mail karger@karger.ch
www.karger.com

0302–2838/01/0399–0013$17.50/0

Accessible online at:
www.karger.com/journals/eur

Dr. H.J. Stoevelaar
Institute for Health Care Policy and Management, Erasmus University
PO Box 1738
NL–3000 DR Rotterdam (The Netherlands)
Tel. +31 10 408 8562, Fax +31 10 408 9092, E-Mail stoevelaar@bmg.eur.nl

useful in complementing evidence-based guidelines for LUTS suggestive of BPO in the grey area of treatment choice.

Introduction

The availability of various new treatments for lower urinary tract symptoms (LUTS) suggestive of benign prostatic obstruction (BPO) or shortly LUTS, necessitates careful consideration of the appropriateness of their use for various patient groups. In this respect, evidence-based medicine (EBM), the application of evidence from valid clinical studies to clinical practice, should be the guiding principle [1].

However, despite the impressive number of studies that have been published over the last decade, there is very often insufficient evidence on which to base clear statements about 'the right treatment for every patient'. Evidence-based guidelines, such as that of the Agency for Health Care Policy and Research (AHCPR, 1994) [2] show a large grey area in which no conclusive evidence exists about the most appropriate treatment choice. As a consequence, the decision making process in daily clinical practice is often based on the personal experience and beliefs of individual doctors. Since thousands of patients are treated each day, this clinical expertise may, at an aggregate level, generate valuable information to complement evidence-based guidelines.

The American research institute RAND, in collaboration with the University of California at Los Angeles, has developed a method (RAM: RAND Appropriateness Method) to systematically canvass clinical expertise to assess the appropriateness of medical and surgical procedures [3]. This modified Delphi procedure has been successfully applied in various fields of medicine [4–7]. Recently, we applied this method in a Dutch study on treatment of LUTS, the results of which revealed consistent opinions on a relatively large proportion of indications in the grey area of treatment choice [8]. In this article, we present the results of an extended study at a supranational level. Urologists from five different European countries participated in an international panel, following the same method as was used by the Dutch panel. This study was undertaken as part of a European program on the appropriate indications of various medical and surgical procedures (BIOMED). The study aims were threefold: (1) to analyse the opinions of experienced European urologists on the appropriate indications for treatment of LUTS in urological practice; (2) to compare the results with those of the Dutch panel study; (3) to assess the potential use of the panel results in further guideline development.

Methods

RAND Appropriateness Method (RAM)

In the RAM [3], a panel of experts is asked to rate the appropriateness of one or more treatments for a systematically constructed set of indications (cases of hypothetical patients). These indications are based on a combination of the various diagnostic variables that are considered to be relevant to treatment choice. A treatment is defined as 'appropriate' for an indication if the expected benefits outweigh the expected negative consequences by a sufficient margin that the treatment is worth performing. Important aspects in this respect are: effectiveness, speed and durability of the effect, extent of invasiveness, ease and discomfort, adverse events and complications. Financial costs are not taken into consideration. The rating process consists of two rounds. In the first round, the panel members individually rate the appropriateness of one or more treatments for each indication, in comparison to another treatment or 'doing nothing'. For that purpose, a 9-point scale is used in which (9) is 'extremely appropriate', (1) is 'extremely inappropriate' and (5) is 'uncertain' or 'neither better nor worse than the alternative treatment'.

After analysis and feedback of the results, the panel convenes in a 1–2 day meeting to discuss the results. The aim of this meeting is not to reach consensus, but to explore differences in the perceptions of definitions used and in the opinions regarding appropriateness. During the meeting, a second rating round takes place in which panellists are given the opportunity to re-rate the indications. Based on the individual ratings, aggregate panel ratings are calculated for each indication (appropriate, inappropriate, and uncertain).

In many RAM studies, the panel results are used as reference values to assess the extent to which appropriate care is provided in daily clinical practice [4–7]. In this study, however, the principal aim was to assess the usefulness of the panel ratings in further guideline development.

Panel Composition

The panel consisted of fifteen European urologists from five different countries (Germany, The Netherlands, Spain, Sweden and The United Kingdom). All panellists had a broad experience in the diagnostic evaluation and treatment of LUTS.

Target Population, Definitions and Criteria

The study was restricted to indications describing patients in the grey area of treatment choice, that is, to patients for whom the AHCPR guideline does not give clear indications for treatment choice. Indications relating to patients with mild symptoms, acute conditions, bladder stones, and those with co-morbidity and/or medication relevant to treatment choice were not employed in the study. Because daily clinical practice was the starting point of this study, only therapies that are commonly available to every urologist in the participating countries were taken into consideration. These were surgery (transurethral resection or incision of the prostate, open prostatectomy), α_1-adrenoceptor antagonists, 5α-reductase-inhibitors (finasteride), and watchful waiting ('no active intervention').

Indication Construction and Rating Lists

In the RAM, each indication corresponds to a hypothetical patient characterised by the values of the diagnostic variables relevant to treatment choice. As was done in the Dutch panel study [8], nine variables were used as the basis for the indication construction. The definitions and cut-off points of these variables are given in table 1. In total, there were 7 variables with 2 categories and 2 variables with 3 categories. The number of possible combinations was therefore 1,152 ($2^7 * 3^2$). In an attempt to reduce the number of indications to be rated, all combinations were examined to detect unrealistic indications. However, no indications were found that could be excluded in advance. The construction of the rating list was based on a tree-like structure, in that the variables formed a hierarchical structure. Using the first variable (previous treatment), the indications were split into two chapters of equal size (1, no previous treatment; 2, failure of α_1-adrenoceptor antagonist treatment). Within each chapter, the remaining variables were further divided. For each indication, the panel members were asked to rate the appropriateness of three active treatments (surgery, α_1-adrenoceptor antagonists, finasteride), each in comparison with the option of watchful waiting, using a 9-point scale. An example of the rating list is given in figure 1. The total rating list consisted of 3,456 ratings (3 treatment comparisons for 1,152 indications).

Preparation of the Rating Round

Before the rating process, the panel members were provided with a review of the literature on the indications for the treatment of LUTS [9]. This overview consisted of an update of the literature study that was used as a basis of the AHCPR practice guideline [2].

Statistical Analysis

The transformation of individual ratings to panel scores was derived from the methodology used in previous RAM studies. Analyses were conducted in two phases. Firstly, the extent of agreement between the panellists was calculated for each indication. For that purpose, the 9-point scale was divided into three sections (1–3; 4–6; 7–9). The criteria for agreement are listed in table 2a. Subsequently, the panel judgements on appropriateness were calculated (see table 2b). The relationship between the diagnostic variables and the appropriateness ratings was studied using logistic regression.

Table 1. Overview of the diagnostic variables used in the construction of indications

	Criteria	Categories
1	Previous treatment	a. No previous active treatment b. Failure of an α_1-adrenoceptor antagonist[1]
2	Age	a. <70 years old b. ≥70 years old
3	Symptom severity	a. Moderate[2] b. Severe[3]
4	Nature of symptoms	a. Not specific[4] b. Predominantly irritative[5]
5	Bothersomeness	a. Acceptable[6] b. Unacceptable[7]
6	Urinary tract infections	a. <2 in previous year b. ≥2 in previous year
7	Urinary peakflow (Q_{max})	a. >15 ml/s b. 10–15 ml/s c. <10 ml/s
8	Prostate size/volume (V_{pros})	a. <30 ml b. 30–50 ml c. >50 ml
9	Postvoid residual urine (PVR)	a. <150 ml b. ≥150 ml

1 The use of an α_1-adrenoceptor antagonist has been stopped due to insufficient therapeutic effect and/or side effects. The previous use of finasteride was not taken into consideration.
2 Comparable to the American Urological Association Symptom Index (AUA-7) score 8–19 [16].
3 Comparable to the AUA-7 score 20–35.
4 Mixed symptoms: not predominantly obstructive or irritative.
5 Frequency and/or nocturia and/or urge constitute the most important symptoms.
6 The patient can, for the time being, tolerate the symptoms.
7 The symptoms are difficult to tolerate.

Results

The first rating round took place in January 1999. The percentage of invalid or missing ratings was low (range 0–1.3%). Strong agreement was found in 42% of indications, while strong disagreement existed in only 1%. The other indications (57%) were considered indeterminate.

The panel convened on March 13, 1999 in Amsterdam. Fourteen of the fifteen panel members attended. Prior to the meeting, the panellists had received an overview of their own ratings, in comparison to the anonymous results of the other panel members. Although the discussion revealed no relevant differences in the interpretation of definitions and procedures used, some comments were made on the variables and cut-off points that were included. Firstly, the panel expressed the view that, given the strong correlation between 'symptom severity' and 'bothersomeness', the inclusion of both variables may be unnecessary. Secondly, it was argued that for patients with 'high flow' (Q_{max} >15 ml/s), the existence of other causes should be considered, particularly in the case of severe symptoms and/or large volumes of postvoid residual urine. Although these conditions were incorporated in the exclusion criteria for this study, it was suggested that such patients are, in general, strongly suspected of having other diseases that require a different diagnostic and therapeutic approach. Because these considerations constituted insufficient reason to change the total indication

Chapter 1		no previous active treatment				Page 1
Age		< 70				
Symptom severity		moderate				
Nature of symptoms		not specific				
Bothersomeness		acceptable				
Urinary tract infections		< 2 in the previous year				
			Surgery	α-blocker	Finasteride	
Q_{max} > 15	V_{pros} < 30	RU < 150	1 2 3 4 5 6 7 8 9	1 2 3 4 5 6 7 8 9	1 2 3 4 5 6 7 8 9	0001 - 0003
		RU ≥ 150	1 2 3 4 5 6 7 8 9	1 2 3 4 5 6 7 8 9	1 2 3 4 5 6 7 8 9	0004 - 0006
	V_{pros} 30-50	RU < 150	1 2 3 4 5 6 7 8 9	1 2 3 4 5 6 7 8 9	1 2 3 4 5 6 7 8 9	0007 - 0009
		RU ≥ 150	1 2 3 4 5 6 7 8 9	1 2 3 4 5 6 7 8 9	1 2 3 4 5 6 7 8 9	0010 - 0012
	V_{pros} > 50	RU < 150	1 2 3 4 5 6 7 8 9	1 2 3 4 5 6 7 8 9	1 2 3 4 5 6 7 8 9	0013 - 0015
		RU ≥ 150	1 2 3 4 5 6 7 8 9	1 2 3 4 5 6 7 8 9	1 2 3 4 5 6 7 8 9	0016 - 0018
Q_{max} 10-15	V_{pros} < 30	RU < 150	1 2 3 4 5 6 7 8 9	1 2 3 4 5 6 7 8 9	1 2 3 4 5 6 7 8 9	0019 - 0021
		RU ≥ 150	1 2 3 4 5 6 7 8 9	1 2 3 4 5 6 7 8 9	1 2 3 4 5 6 7 8 9	0022 - 0024
	V_{pros} 30-50	RU < 150	1 2 3 4 5 6 7 8 9	1 2 3 4 5 6 7 8 9	1 2 3 4 5 6 7 8 9	0025 - 0027
		RU ≥ 150	1 2 3 4 5 6 7 8 9	1 2 3 4 5 6 7 8 9	1 2 3 4 5 6 7 8 9	0028 - 0030
	V_{pros} > 50	RU < 150	1 2 3 4 5 6 7 8 9	1 2 3 4 5 6 7 8 9	1 2 3 4 5 6 7 8 9	0031 - 0033
		RU ≥ 150	1 2 3 4 5 6 7 8 9	1 2 3 4 5 6 7 8 9	1 2 3 4 5 6 7 8 9	0034 - 0036
1 = much worse than watchful waiting			5 - neither better nor worse than watchful waiting		9 = much better than watchful waiting	

Fig. 1. Example of the rating list.

Table 2. Criteria for agreement (A) and appropriateness (B)

	Category	Description
A	Agreement	≤4 individual scores outside the section in which the median score fell
	Disagreement	≥5 individual scores in each of the sections 1–3 and 7–9
	Indeterminate	All other outcomes
B	Appropriate	The median score lies in section 7–9 without disagreement of the panel members
	Inappropriate	The median score lies in section 1–3 without disagreement of the panel members
	Uncertain	All other outcomes

structure, it was decided to maintain the original list for the second rating round. The re-ratings were restricted to: (1) the first 54 indications, in order to eliminate the impact of any learning process; (2) indications for which disagreement existed in the first round; (3) indications for which varying only one characteristic led to disagreement. The second rating round was held during the panel meeting. The panellist who was absent carried out the re-ratings later. As a result of the revisions, the percentage of indications for which disagreement existed decreased to almost zero (see table 3). The key figures on the appropriateness assessment are given in table 4. In more than half the indications in chapter 1 (no previous active treatment), an α_1-adrenoceptor antagonist was considered appropriate as the (initial) treatment. Surgery took second place while finasteride was judged to be appropriate in only a small percentage of the indications. This type of medication also showed the most pronounced contra-indications (inappropriate indications). Almost all these indications (95%) concerned patients with small prostate volumes (<30 ml). For indications in which α_1-adrenoceptor antagonist treatment had failed (chapter 2), surgery was most frequently reported as an appropriate therapy. The panel considered the prescription of another type of α_1-adrenoceptor antagonist inappropriate for all of these indications. The figures for finasteride were almost identical to those of chapter 1.

The relationship between the various diagnostic variables and the panel judgement 'appropriate' was examined using logistic regression analysis. In general, strong and consistent results were found. A reduced peakflow increased the probability of all active treatments more than any other single factor. Severe symptoms, unacceptable bother, recurrent urinary tract infections and large residual urine volume increased the likelihood of both surgery and α_1-adrenoceptor antagonist treatment, while the use of finasteride was strongly linked to a greatly enlarged prostate. Patients with predominantly irritative symptoms were more likely to receive an α_1-adrenoceptor antagonist than surgery. Because no meaningful interactions were found, the impact of the variables was merely cumulative: the indications for surgery and α_1-adrenoceptor antagonists were strongly associated with the number of unfavourable diagnostic conditions (see fig. 2). The results on finasteride should be considered with caution, because the number of appropriate indications for this type of medication was rather small. Except for α_1-adrenoceptor antagonist treatment (no regression analysis was possible because all indications were judged to be inappropriate), the analysis on chapter 2 showed comparable patterns for surgery and finasteride.

Comparison with Dutch Panel Results

As mentioned in the introduction, this European study followed exactly the same procedure as was used in a recent panel study in the Netherlands. The European

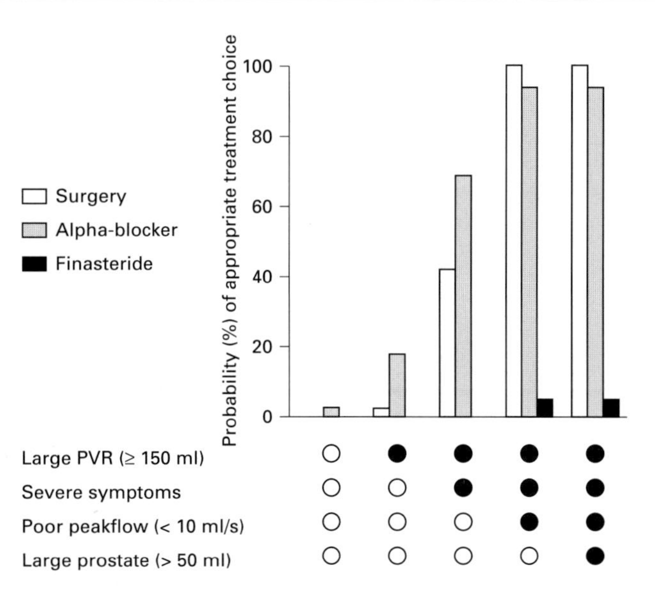

Fig. 2. Example of the cumulative effect of diagnostic variables on the panel judgement 'appropriate' for surgery, α-blockers and finasteride. Probabilities based on logistic regression. The reference patient (4 hollow bullets on the left) is defined as follows: no previous active intervention, age <70 years, no specific symptoms, acceptable bother, urinary tract infections <2 in the previous year, peakflow 10–15 ml/s, prostate volume 30–50 ml, postvoid residual urine <150 ml.

Table 3. Agreement among the panel members after the second rating round (percentages); sum of row totals is 100%

Chapter	Agreement	Indeterminate	Disagreement
No previous treatment	27.5	72.3	0.2
Failure of an α_1-adrenoceptor antagonist	57.4	42.5	0.1
Total	42.5	57.4	0.1

Table 4. Appropriateness ratings after the second round (percentages); sum of row totals is 100%

Chapter/treatment	Appropriate	Uncertain	Inappropriate
Chapter 1: No previous treatment			
Surgery	44.4	46.7	8.9
α_1-Adrenoceptor antagonists	55.9	44.1	0.0
Finasteride	6.4	62.5	31.1
Chapter 2: Failure of an α_1-adrenoceptor antagonist			
Surgery	57.3	41.1	1.6
Other type of α_1-adrenoceptor antagonist	0.0	0.0	100.0
Finasteride	7.5	58.5	34.0

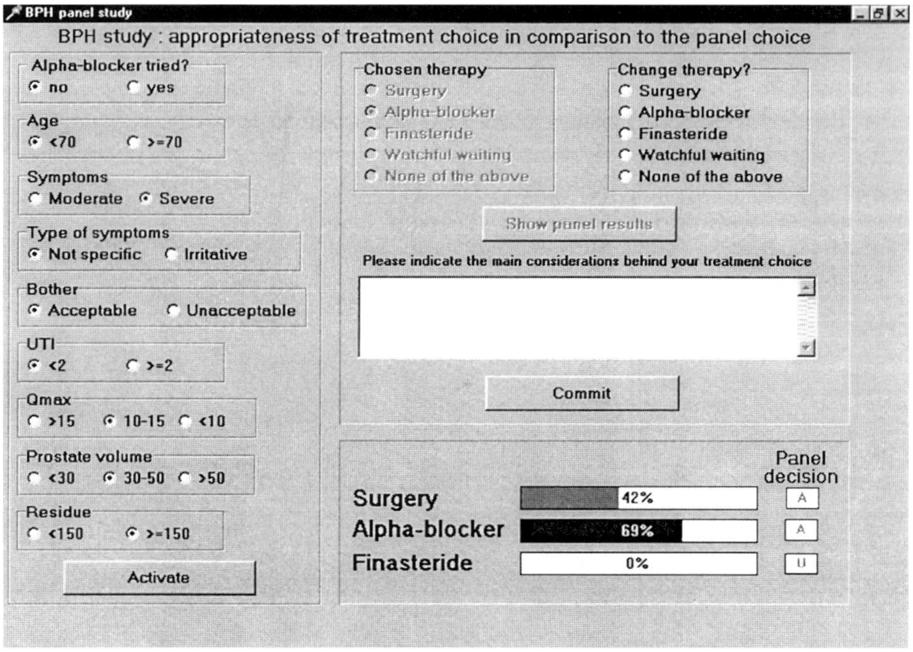

Fig. 3. User interface of the decision support program.

panel consisted of 15 urologists as opposed to 12 in the Dutch. Comparison of the European and Dutch data (detailed report published separately) [10], showed consistent and highly similar patterns. The mean scores (9-point scale) were identical in 41% of the 3,456 ratings, and in 99% the difference was at most 2 points. The overall agreement on the appropriateness judgements was 84% (kappa value 0.76).

Use of Panel Results in Guideline Development

As supported by the consistent panel results, clinical expertise may generate a useful contribution to further guideline development where evidence from clinical studies is lacking. However, given the large number of diagnostic variables, each making its own contribution, it is not easy to translate the panel results into comprehensive and convenient written recommendations. Therefore, we developed a computer program to facilitate the use and evaluation of the appropriateness data in daily clinical practice. Figure 3 shows the user interface. On the left side, the diagnostic patient characteristics can be selected. The user then indicates the initial treatment choice. Subsequently the panel recommendations are given in two forms. Text boxes indicate the actual ratings for that indication while the coloured gauges express the results of the logistic regression analysis over all indications. This analysis seeks to determine the underlying pattern of contributions made by the variables, uncontaminated by 'random noise' at the individual indication level. The values depicted in these gauges represent the probability that the panel would consider the treatments as being appropriate, each in comparison to the option of watchful waiting, if the rating process were to be carried out again. After the panel recommendations are shown, the urologist is offered the opportunity to change his decision and to document the principal considerations for treatment choice in this patient. All data, including potential changes in treatment choice, are automatically stored in a database. This database enables the evaluation and validation of the program in clinical studies and in daily practice. Future research will examine the value of this decision aid.

Discussion

The RAND Appropriateness Method was used to systematically investigate the opinions of a panel of urologists on the appropriate treatment of LUTS. The study focussed on patients for which the AHCPR guideline [2] does not provide clear indications for treatment choice. Overall, there was a considerable extent of agreement between the panellists. Moreover, logistic regression analysis revealed strong and consistent associations between the diagnostic variables included and the final panel judgements. The results indicate that treatment choice is determined by the sum of 'unfavourable' diagnostic characteristics with different weights, and not by particular combinations. Because the appropriateness of all active treatments was compared to the option of 'watchful waiting', conclusions on the extent of appropriateness between pairs treatments can only be drawn indirectly. Additional analyses are needed to refine the recommendations on the relative appropriateness among the various treatments.

The usefulness of the panel results depends on the validity and reliability of the panel method on the one hand, and their applicability in daily clinical practice on the other hand. The external validity of this model is supported by the large extent of agreement we found between the results of this study and an essentially identical Dutch panel study [8, 10]. Other methodological aspects of the RAM have been extensively tested in various studies and show, in general, consistent results [4, 11–15].

Nevertheless, the principal limitation lies in the subjectivity of the panel opinions, and their validity should be evaluated in clinical studies. The function of the panel recommendations is therefore restricted to that of a 'professional mirror': urologists are offered the opportunity to compare their own treatment decisions to the opinion of a panel of experienced colleagues.

The applicability of the panel results in daily clinical practice is complicated by the large number of variables included. Therefore, the use of a computer program as a decision aid appears to be essential. In combination with a database, this program also enables the evaluation of the clinical relevance of the patient profiles included.

Conclusions

Given the relatively large extent of agreement and the consistency of the panel data, the results may be useful in complementing evidence-based guidelines in the grey area of treatment choice. However, the validity and clinical applicability of the panel recommendations should be tested in further studies.

Acknowledgements

This study has been carried out as part of the Concerted Action 'A method to integrate scientific and clinical knowledge to achieve the appropriate utilisation of major medical and surgical procedures', financed by Directorate General XII of the European Commission under the BIOMED II program (contract no. BMH4-CT96-0212).

References

1 Speakman MJ: Lower urinary tract symptoms suggestive of benign prostatic obstruction: What is the available evidence for rational management? Eur Urol 2001;39(suppl 3):6–12.

2 McConnell JD, Barry MJ, Bruskewitz RC, Bueschen AJ, Denton SE, Holtgrewe HL, Lange JL, McClennan BL, Mebust WK, Reilly NJ, Roberts RG, Sacks SA, Wasson JH: Benign prostatic hyperplasia: Diagnosis and treatment. Clinical practice guideline, number 8. AHCPR publication no. 94-0582. Rockville, MD: Agency for Health Care Policy and Research, Public Health Service, US Department of Health and Human Services, 1994.

3 Kahn KL, Kosecoff J, Chassin MR, Flynn MF, Fink A, Pattaphongse N, Solomon DH, Brook RH: Measuring the clinical appropriateness of the use of a procedure. Can we do it? Med Care 1988;26:415–422.

4 Park RE, Fink A, Brook RH, Chassin MR, Kahn KL, Merrick NJ, Kosecoff J, Solomon DH: Physician ratings of appropriate indications for six medical and surgical procedures. Am J Publ Health 1986;76:766–772.

5 Hilborne LH, Leape LL, Bernstein SJ, Park RE, Fiske ME, Kamberg CJ, Pindar Roth C, Brook RH: The appropriateness of use of percutaneous transluminal coronary angioplasty in New York State. JAMA 1993;269:761–765.

6 Tobacman JK, Lee P, Zimmerman B, Kolder H, Hilborne L, Brook RH: Assessment of appropriateness of cataract surgery at ten academic medical centers in 1990. Ophthalmology 1996;103:207–215.

7 Larequi-Lauber T, Vader JP, Burnand B, Brook RH, Kosecoff J, Sloutskis D, Frankhauser H, Berney J, De Tribolet N, Paccaud F: Appropriateness of indications for surgery of lumbar disc hernia and spinal stenosis. Spine 1997;22:203–209.

8 Stoevelaar HJ, McDonnell J, Van de Beek C, Casparie AF: Appropriate treatment of benign prostatic hyperplasia: enhancing the indication for treatment by systematic analysis of expert opinion. Ned Tijdschr Geneeskd 1999;48: 2425–2429.

9 Stoevelaar HJ, Redekop WK: Treatment of benign prostatic hyperplasia: An update of the AHCPR clinical practice guideline. Rotterdam, Institute for Health Care Policy and Management (Erasmus University), 1998.

10 McDonnell J, Stoevelaar HJ, Bosch JLHR, Kahan JP, Dutch and European Panels on the Appropriate Treatment of BPH: The appropriateness of treatment of benign prostatic hyperplasia: A comparison of Dutch and multinational criteria. Health Policy (accepted for publication).

11 McClellan M, Brook RH: Appropriateness of care: Comparison of global and outcome methods to set standards. Med Care 1992;30:565–586.

12 McDonnell J, Meijler A, Kahan JP, Bernstein SJ, Rigter H: Panellist consistency in the assessment of medical appropriateness. Health Policy 1996;37:139–152.

13 Vader JP, Burnand B, Froehlich F, Dupriez K, Larequi-Lauber T, Pache I, Dubois RW, Gonvers JJ, Brook RH: Appropriateness of upper gastrointestinal endoscopy: Comparison of American and Swiss criteria. Int J Qual Health Care 1997;9:87–92.

14 Burnand B, Vader JP, Froehlich F, Dupriez K, Larequi-Lauber T, Pache I, Dubois RW, Brook RH, Gonvers JJ: Reliability of panel-based guidelines for colonoscopy: An international comparison. Gastrointest Endosc1998;47:162–166.

15 Shekelle PG, Kahan JP, Bernstein SJ, Leape LL, Kamberg CJ, Park RE: The reproducibility of a method to identify the overuse and underuse of medical procedures. N Engl J Med 1998;338:1888–1895.

16 Barry MJ, Fowler FJ Jr, O'Leary MP, Bruskewitz RC, Holtgrewe HL, Mebust WK, Cockett AT: The American Urological Association symptom index for benign prostatic hyperplasia. J Urol 1992;148:1549–1557.

European Urology

Eur Urol 2001;39(suppl 3):20–25

Lower Urinary Tract Symptoms Suggestive of Benign Prostatic Obstruction – What's the Long-Term Effectiveness of Medical Therapies?

Martin C. Michel   Mark Goepel

Department of Medicine and Urology, University of Essen, Essen, Germany

Key Words

Acute urinary retention · Progression to surgery · Benign prostatic obstruction · α_1-Adrenoceptor antagonists · Finasteride · Long-term · Disease progression

Abstract

The primary treatment goal in patients with lower urinary tract symptoms (LUTS) suggestive of benign prostatic obstruction (BPO) is symptom relief. However, it is also important to assess the effects of medical treatments on disease progression because this can lead to complications such as acute urinary retention or can ultimately require surgical treatment. In a placebo-controlled study finasteride was shown to reduce the incidence of acute urinary retention and the need for surgery in patients with LUTS suggestive of BPO. While α_1-adrenoceptor antagonists are superior to finasteride with regard to LUTS relief, systematic studies on their effects on BPO complications and progression to surgery are not available. However, we reviewed a number of smaller studies which consistently indicate that α_1-adrenoceptor antagonists may be at least as effective as finasteride in the prevention of acute urinary retention or the need for surgery in patients with LUTS suggestive of BPO. While this needs to be confirmed in adequately designed and powered studies, such evidence should be taken into consideration when choosing between α_1-adrenoceptor antagonists and finasteride treatment.

Introduction

Lower urinary tract symptoms (LUTS) suggestive of benign prostatic obstruction (BPO) are a disease state which increases in elderly males. At present multiple medical and surgical treatment options are available for such patients, but the specific advantages and disadvantages of the various options relative to others, particularly with regard to long-term treatment outcomes, are not well known in many cases. In this review we will compare the two main forms of rational medical treatment, i.e. α_1-adrenoceptor antagonists and finasteride, with regard to their effects on BPO complications and disease progression.

Treatment Effects on LUTS

Rapid symptom relief is the key reason to seek treatment for most patients with LUTS suggestive of BPO. While α_1-adrenoceptor antagonists reduce LUTS within days or weeks, finasteride requires several months to achieve symptom relief [1]. To compare the efficacy of finasteride and the α_1-adrenoceptor antagonists, three double-blind, randomised controlled trials (RCTs) lasting 6–12 months have been performed using terazosin [2], alfuzosin [3] or doxazosin [4] as the α_1-adrenoceptor antagonist (fig. 1). In each study, the α_1-adrenoceptor antagonist lowered I-PSS significantly more than finasteride and, where applicable, than placebo. In contrast, finasteride did not cause a statistically significant greater

KARGER

Fax + 41 61 306 12 34
E-Mail karger@karger.ch
www.karger.com

0302–2838/01/0399–0020$17.50/0

Accessible online at:
www.karger.com/journals/eur

Dr. Martin C. Michel
Nephrol. Lab. IG 1, Klinikum Essen
Hufelandstrasse 55
D–45122 Essen (Germany)
Tel. +49 201 723 4467, Fax +49 201 723 5963, E-Mail martin.michel@uni-essen.de

I-PSS reduction than placebo in these studies. Similar data were seen for urinary flow rates. The apparent lack of effect of finasteride in these studies appears to relate to prostate size of participating patients since a meta-analysis has shown that patients are only likely to benefit from finasteride relative to placebo treatment if baseline prostate volume exceeds 40 ml [5]. In contrast, α_1-adrenoceptor with antagonists work equally well in patients small or large prostates [6] and with mild, moderate or severe LUTS suggestive of BPO [7]. Based on these data it appears that α_1-adrenoceptor antagonists are preferable to finasteride in the treatment of LUTS suggestive of BPO due to a faster onset of symptom relief and a greater extent of symptom relief during treatment. This conclusion is also supported by circumstantial evidence from several real life practice studies [8, 9, 10]. Interestingly, data from randomised direct comparative studies indicate that finasteride is equally effective as saw palmetto extracts [11, 12], and accordingly real life practice studies [9] and limited randomised direct comparative studies [13] have reported α_1-adrenoceptor antagonists to be more effective than plant extracts, at least in the short-term.

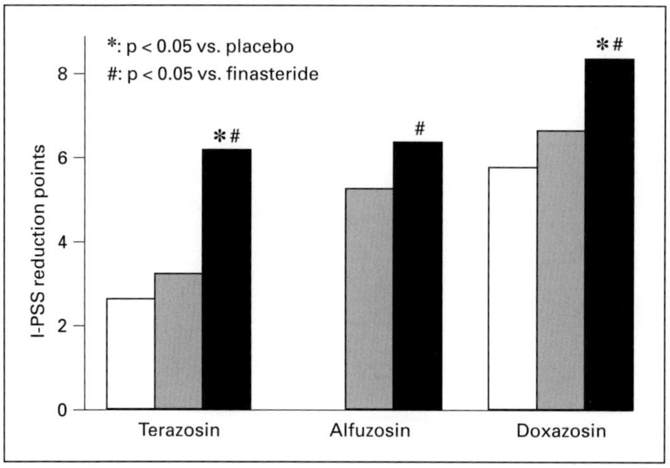

Fig. 1. Effect of placebo (open bars), finasteride (hatched bars) or an α_1-adrenoceptor antagonist (filled bars) on I-PSS in three studies using terazosin (VA study), alfuzosin (ALFIN) or doxazosin (PREDICT) as the α_1-adrenoceptor antagonist. Adapted from [2, 3, 4].

Natural History of LUTS Suggestive of BPO

The prevalence and average severity of LUTS suggestive of BPO in the population increase with age [14, 15]. The disease course in an individual patient, however, is difficult to predict. For example, a 4-year follow-up of 500 candidates for elective prostatectomy treated non-operatively found that among men with moderate symptoms 1/4 eventually underwent prostatectomy, 1/8 had progression to severe symptoms without undergoing surgery, 1/2 remained stable with moderate symptoms and 1/8 even had improvement to only mild symptoms [16]. In another study, a major fraction of patients with LUTS and benign prostatic enlargement but without urodynamically detectable bladder obstruction showed symptom improvement during a 6-month period of watchful waiting [17]. Thus, symptoms abate without treatment in some patients, but more patients experience an increase in symptom severity over time. Accordingly, one study demonstrates an increase in mean LUTS with age, and within each decade of patients the group mean symptom score clearly increases over the next 5 years [18]. Accordingly, approximately 2.5% of patients with mild LUTS suggestive of BPO receiving watchful waiting [16] or placebo treatment [19] will require surgery each year; when LUTS are moderate or severe, the yearly incidence of progression to surgery during watchful waiting may increase to 6% or almost 10% per year, respectively [16].

Nowadays LUTS suggestive of BPO primarily affect quality of life and in contrast to diseases such as arterial hypertension, cause only relatively little morbidity or mortality. Several decades ago, however, benign prostatic hyperplasia caused mortality in a significant number of cases, e.g. through renal failure, urological infections and, most commonly, surgical treatment but this mortality has markedly decreased in the last four decades [20]. Nevertheless, LUTS suggestive of BPO remains a chronically progressive disease which can lead to complications such as acute urinary retention (AUR), recurrent urinary tract infections, bladder stones and renal dysfunction. In a 4-year follow-up of 500 candidates for elective prostatectomy treated non-operatively [16] as well as in 1,503 patients treated with placebo for 4 years as part of the PLESS study [19], the AUR risk was approximately 2.5% per year. Long-term changes in flow rates and symptoms [21] as well as occurrence of AUR [22] are best predicted by serum levels of prostate-specific antigen at baseline.

Effects of Medical Treatment on Acute Urinary Retention

While patients primarily seek treatment for LUTS suggestive of BPO to receive symptom relief, prevention of disease progression, manifested as development of disease complications and/or switch to other medical or surgical

Table 1. Effect of placebo, finasteride or an α_1-adrenoceptor antagonist on the incidence of acute urinary retention

Study	Placebo	Finasteride	α_1-Adrenoceptor antagonist
Jardin et al., 1991 [25]	5.24 (7/134)	n.s.	0.80* (1/126, alfuzosin)
McConnell et al., 1998 [19]	2.40 (36/1,503)	0.93* (14/1,513)	n.s.
Debruyne et al., 1998 [3]	n.s.	0.58 (1/172)	1.12 (2/179, alfuzosin)
Kirby et al., 1999 [4]	1.59 (4/252)	1.27 (3/237)	0.0 (0/249, doxazosin)
Michel et al., 1999 [26]	n.s.	n.s.	0.49 (4/811, tamsulosin)

Data are cases per 100 patient years with the total number of cases and patient years in parentheses. * $p < 0.05$ vs. placebo within that study; n.s. = not studied.

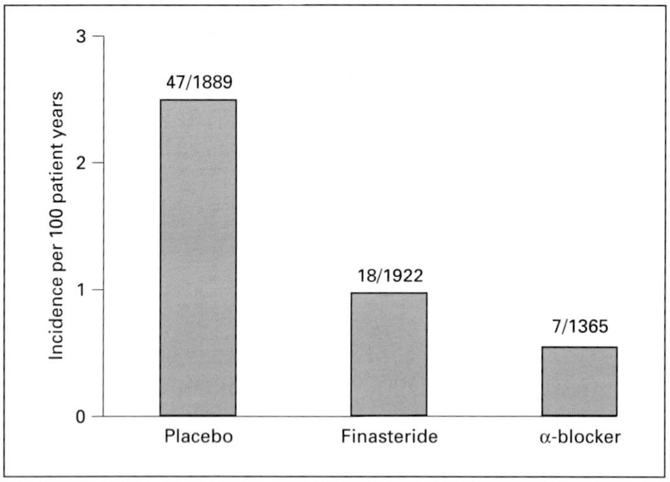

Fig. 2. Effect of placebo, finasteride or an α_1-adrenoceptor antagonist on the incidence of acute urinary retention expressed as cases per 100 patient years. Data are pooled afflicted patients and patient years from [3, 4, 19, 25, 26]. Total number of cases and patient years for each agent are shown above the individual bars. Data from the individual studies are shown in table 1.

therapies, is certainly an important treatment goal. In this context it should be considered that the average patient initially receiving medical treatment of LUTS suggestive of BPO is in his early to mid-sixties [23, 24]. This implies a remaining life expectancy of 15–20 years in developed countries. Treatment results over this extended period are the ultimate yard stick to judge treatment modalities in patients with LUTS suggestive of BPO, but unfortunately are not available for any form of treatment. Therefore, the impact of treatment on disease progression must be weighed against the achievable extent of symptom relief to choose optimal treatment for a given patient. Given the dominance of disease-induced quality of life reduction vs. disease-induced morbidity and mortality, excellent tolerability becomes an additional criterion in treatment selection.

A recent landmark study (PLESS) has compared the effect of randomised, double-blind finasteride and placebo treatment on the incidence of AUR in a group of 3,040 men with LUTS suggestive of BPO followed for a period of 4 years [19]. While 99 of 1,503 placebo-treated patients (7%) experienced one or more AUR episodes, only 42 out of 1,513 finasteride-treated patients (3%) developed AUR. This reduction in incidence was similar for spontaneous and precipitated AUR. In this context it is interesting, that prostate volume, which was measured in approximately 10% of patients, gradually increased with time in placebo-treated patients by up to 15%, while it declined by almost 20% during the first year in finasteride-treated patients and remained at that level for the remaining observational period. Despite the gradual increase in prostate size in the placebo-treated patients, symptom score and urine flow rates remained stable between 1 and 4 years. In contrast, symptom scores and flow rates tended to improve over the entire observational period in the finasteride group.

Whether α_1-adrenoceptor antagonists also lower AUR incidence and/or prevent other BPO complications, has not been sufficiently studied. For the practicing physician, this creates a therapeutic dilemma, i.e. whether to use finasteride because of proven prevention of disease complications or an α_1-adrenoceptor antagonist because of faster and greater symptom relief. Therefore, we have retrospectively analysed published studies which lasted at least 6 months, were performed according to Good Clinical Practice (GCP) guidelines and reported on the incidence of AUR. We have identified five such studies [3, 4, 19, 25, 26]. Results from the individual studies are shown in table 1, a pooled analysis of the data is shown in figure 2. From this comparison it appears that treatment with an α_1-adrenoceptor antagonist lowers AUR incidence at least as much as finasteride treatment. Although the reduction of AUR incidence by α_1-adrenoceptor antagonists reached statistical significance in one study, in which the incidence in the placebo arm had been high [25], our analysis can be criticised for several reasons. None of the α_1-adrenoceptor studies had been designed or powered to test for alterations in the rate of AUR. Accordingly, the α_1-adrenoceptor studies lasted only 6–12 months, whereas the PLESS study lasted 4 years; to account for that, only the data from the first 12 months of the PLESS study were entered into the present analysis to improve study homogeneity. With one exception, the α_1-adrenoceptor studies had much smaller patient numbers than the PLESS study. Finally, some of the α_1-adrenoceptor antagonist studies did not have a placebo arm. All of these criticisms are well taken and clearly indicate that our analysis cannot substitute for a direct comparative study (preferably including a placebo arm) which is designed and powered to look at AUR incidence with the various treatment modalities. Such a study, named MTOPS, is presently underway in the US, but the results are not expected to become available for several years. In the meantime, physicians still have to decide whether to go for faster and greater symptom relief using an α_1-adrenoceptor antagonist or proven slowing of disease progression by finasteride. We feel that in this situation the above data can be taken as circumstantial evidence for the following reasons: Firstly, age, symptom severity, prostate-specific antigen level and prostate size are statistical predictors of AUR incidence, with the latter two being most predictive [16, 19, 22], and where reported these parameters were very similar in all five studies. Second, although some of the α_1-adrenoceptor studies did not have a placebo arm, an event such as AUR is unlikely to be recorded in a falsely positive or negative manner in a study according to GCP guidelines; hence even studies without a placebo arm can contribute valuable information to the overall analysis. Third, the incidence of AUR in the placebo arms of PLESS, the two α_1-adrenoceptor antagonist studies and a previous study on watchful waiting [27] overall are in reasonable agreement and in each case are higher than in any of the active treatment arms with finasteride or α_1-adrenoceptor antagonists. Fourth, although the α_1-adrenoceptor antagonist studies had only small finasteride arms, the AUR incidence in those finasteride arms was almost identical with that in PLESS. Fifth, the incidence in the α_1-adrenoceptor antagonist arms was very similar across all studies and in no case higher than in the lowest placebo arm of any study. Sixth, in one study α_1-adrenoceptor antagonist treatment was associated with a significantly lower AUR incidence than placebo. Finally, two other lines of evidence also indicate that treatment with α_1-adrenoceptor antagonists may prevent AUR. In one study the percentage of patients with AUR being able to void successfully after removal of the catheter was almost twice as high in those treated with the α_1-adrenoceptor antagonist alfuzosin than in those with placebo [28]. Moreover, neoadjuvant treatment with the α_1-adrenoceptor antagonist tamsulosin in patients undergoing thermotherapy for LUTS suggestive of BPO reduced the AUR rate in those patients from 12% to 2% [29]. Based on these data we propose that in the absence of results from a definitive study our analysis can be taken as preliminary evidence to indicate that α_1-adrenoceptor antagonists may have a similar beneficial effect on AUR incidence as finasteride. The difference between the observed AUR incidences during α_1-adrenoceptor antagonist and finasteride treatment, however, are too small to be interpreted in a meaningful way. Whether the reduction of AUR incidence also extends to a reduced incidence of other BPO complications such as recurrent urinary tract infections, bladder stones and renal dysfunction remains to be determined for finasteride and the α_1-adrenoceptor antagonists.

Effects of Medical Treatment on Progression to Surgery

Another facet of disease progression is the observation that approximately 2.5% of patients with mild LUTS suggestive of BPO receiving watchful waiting [16] or placebo treatment [19] will require surgery each year, with up to 6% or almost 10% in patients with moderate or severe symptoms [16]. In this regard the risk for surgery is associated with the disease severity, specifically serum levels of prostate-specific antigen, at baseline [16, 22]. Therefore, it is a major concern with all forms of medical treatment that disease severity may increase with time despite treatment and reach a point where surgery becomes inevitable. Given a typical age of early to mid-sixties at the beginning of medical treatment [23, 24] and a remaining life expectancy of 15–20 years, this poses the risk of deferring the need for surgical treatment to an age where the patient is more likely to experience adverse effects of surgery.

In this regard the PLESS study has demonstrated that a 4-year treatment with finasteride relative to placebo reduces the incidence of surgery from 152 cases in 1,503 patients (10%) to 69 cases in 1,513 patients (5%) [19]. α_1-Adrenoceptor antagonists have not been systematically studied in that regard but limited conclusions can be drawn from the PREDICT study [4]. That study was

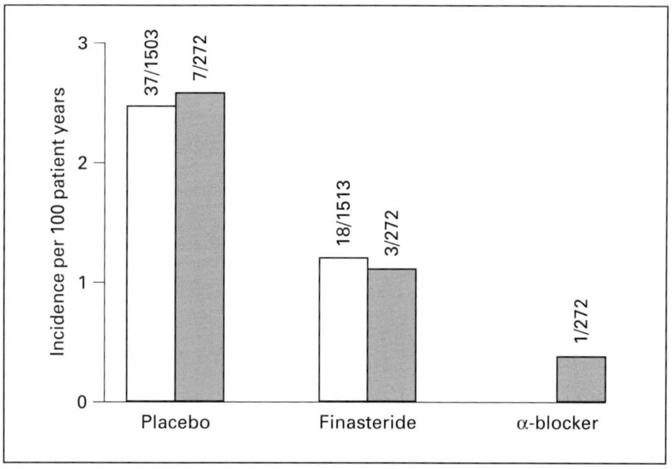

Fig. 3. Effect of placebo, finasteride or an α_1-adrenoceptor antagonist on the incidence of progression to surgery expressed as cases per 100 patient years. Adapted from the PLESS (open bars) and PREDICT (hatched bars) studies [4, 19]. Total number of cases and patient years for each agent are shown above the individual bars.

designed to compare the effects of placebo, finasteride and an α_1-adrenoceptor antagonist on symptom relief during a 1-year treatment. While the study was neither designed nor powered to look at alterations in disease progression, it is interesting that the surgery rates in the placebo and finasteride arms of PREDICT were almost identical to those in PLESS, and that the α_1-adrenoceptor antagonist arm tended to have even lower surgery rates (Fig. 3). With all the caveats discussed above with regard to AUR alterations by α_1-adrenoceptor antagonists, these data indicate that it may be possible that α_1-adrenoceptor antagonists decrease the need for surgery in patients with LUTS suggestive of BPO.

A disease-modifying effect of α_1-adrenoceptor antagonists may be considered surprising since this class of drugs is generally believed to act by smooth muscle relaxation rather than by altering cellular growth, but a number of recent findings challenge this view [30]. Thus, α_1-adrenoceptor agonists cause cellular growth stimulation in many cell types including rat cardiomyocytes [31], canine renal tubular cells [32] and rat arterial smooth muscle cells [33]. A flip side of cellular proliferation is programmed cell death, also known as apoptosis [34]. α_1-Adrenoceptor agonists can prevent apoptosis in non-prostatic cells [35] and correspondingly α_1-adrenoceptor antagonists were reported to increase apoptosis in prostates of patients with LUTS suggestive of BPO [36,37] as it has been reported with androgen ablation [38]. While it should be emphasised that the clinical relevance of these findings remains to be established and that it may be over-optimistic to expect prostate shrinkage upon α_1-adrenoceptor antagonist treatment, these experimental data are in line with the above circumstantial evidence for a disease slowing effect of α_1-adrenoceptor antagonists.

Conclusions and Open Questions

Taken together the available clinical and experimental data indicate that superior symptom relief can be achieved by the α_1-adrenoceptor antagonists without sacrificing the benefit of slowed disease progression, which hitherto has been associated only with finasteride. However, a specific study designed and powered to address these questions (e.g. the MTOPS study) remains necessary and currently is underway. On the other hand, classical RCTs may not fully answer the clinically relevant questions since they hardly can cover the 15–20 years during which a patient may require treatment of LUTS suggestive of BPO. Epidemiological studies looking at indicators of overall patient satisfaction with treatment such as switch to other therapies and at surgery rates among medically treated patients may provide an important additional source of evidence to allow a rational choice between the available forms of medical treatment.

Acknowledgements:

Work in the authors' laboratories was supported by grants from the Deutsche Forschungsgemeinschaft (Go 874/1-1), Boehringer Ingelheim and Yamanouchi.

References

1 Geller J, Kirschenbaum A, Lepor H, Levine AC: Therapeutic controversies: Clinical treatment of benign prostatic hyperplasia. J Clin Endocrinol Metab 1995;80:745–756.

2 Lepor H, Williford WO, Barry MJ, Brawer MK, Dixon CM, Gormley G, Haakenson C, Machi M, Narayan P, Padley RJ: The efficacy of terazosin, finasteride, or both in benign prostatic hyperplasia. New Engl J Med 1996;335:533–539.

3 Debruyne FM, Jardin A, Colloi D, Resel L, Witjes WP, Delauche-Cavallier MC, McCarthy C, Geffriaud-Ricouard C: Sustained-release alfuzosin, finasteride and the combination of both in the treatment of benign prostatic hyperplasia. European ALFIN Study Group. Eur Urol 1998;34:169–175.

4 Kirby R, Altwein JE, Bartsch G, Boyle P, Jardin A, Roehrborn CG: Results of the PREDICT (Prospective European Doxazosin and Combination Therapy) trial. J Urol 1999;161 (suppl):266 (abstract 1027).
5 Boyle P, Gould AL, Roehrborn CG: Prostate volume predicts outcome of treatment of benign prostatic hyperplasia with finasteride: Meta-analysis of randomized clinical trials. Urology 1996;48:398–405.
6 Lepor H, Williford WO, Barry MJ, Haakenson C, Jones K: The impact of medical therapy on bother due to symptoms, quality of life and global outcome, and factors predicting response. Veterans Affairs Cooperative Studies Benign Prostatic Hyperplasia Study Group. J Urol 1998;160:1358–1367.
7 Michel MC, Mehlburger L, Bressel H-U, Goepel M: Comparison of tamsulosin efficacy in subgroups of patients with lower urinary tract symptoms. Prostate Cancer Prost Dis 1998;1: 332–335.
8 Wilton L, Pearce G, Edet E, Freemantle S, Stephens MDB, Mann RD: The safety of finasteride used in benign prostatic hypertrophy: A non-interventional observational cohort study in 14772 patients. Br J Urol 1996;78:379–384.
9 Michel MC, Bressel H-U, Mehlburger L, Goepel M: Tamsulosin: Real life clinical experience in 19,365 patients. Eur Urol 1998;34 (suppl 2): 37–45.
10 Mann RD, Biswas P, Freemantle S, Pearce G, Wilton L: The pharmacovigilance of tamsulosin: Event data on 12484 patients. BJU Int 2000;85:446–450.
11 Carraro J-C, Raynaud J-P, Koch G, Chisholm GD, Di Silverio F, Teillac P, Da Silva FC, Cauquil J, Chopin DK, Hamdy FC, Hanus M, Hauri D, Kalinteris A, Marencak J, Perier A, Perrin P: Comparison of phytotherapy (Permixon) with finasteride in the treatment of benign prostate hyperplasia: A randomized international study of 1,098 patients. Prostate 1996;29:231–240.
12 Sökeland J, Albrecht J: Kombination aus Sabal- und Urticaextrakt vs. Finasterid bei BPH (Stad. I bis II nach Alken). Vergleich der therapeutischen Wirksamkeit in einer einjährigen Doppelblindstudie. Urologe A 1997;36:327–333.
13 Grasso M, Montesano A, Buonaguldi A, Castelli M, Lania C, Rigatti P, Rocco F, Cesana BM, Borghi C: Comparative effects of alfuzosin versus Serenoa repens in the treatment of symptomatic benign prostatic hyperplasia. Arch Esp Urol 1995;48:97–104.
14 Girman CJ, Jacobsen SJ, Guess HA, Oesterling JE, Chute CG, Panser LA, Lieber MM: Natural history of prostatism: Relationship among symptoms, prostate volume and peak urinary flow rate. J Urol 1995;153:1510–1515.
15 Michel MC, Mehlburger L, Schumacher H, Bressel H-U, Goepel M: Effect of diabetes on lower urinary tract symptoms in patients with benign prostatic hyperplasia. J Urol 2000;163: 1725–1729.
16 Barry MJ, Fowler FJjr, Bin L, Pitts JCI, Harris CJ, Mulley AGjr: The natural history of patients with benign prostatic hyperplasia as diagnosed by North American urologists. J Urol 1997;157:10–15.
17 Witjes WPJ, de Wildt MJAM, Rosier PFWM, Caris CTM, Debruyne FMJ, de la Rosette JJMCH: Variability of clinical and pressure-flow study variables after 6 months of watchful waiting in patients with lower urinary tract symptoms and benign prostatic enlargement. J Urol 1996;156:1026–1034.
18 Lee AJ, Garraway WM, Simpson RJ, Fisher W, King D: The natural history of untreated lower urinary tract symptoms in middle-aged and elderly men over a period of five years. Eur Urol 1998;34:325–332.
19 McConnell JD, Bruskewitz R, Walsh P, Andirole G, Lieber M, Holtgrewe HL, Albertsen P, Roehrborn CG, Nickel JC, Want DZ, Taylor AM, Waldstreicher J: The effect of finasteride on the risk of acute urinary retention and the need for surgical treatment among men with benign prostatic hyperplasia. New Engl J Med 1998;338:557–563.
20 Boyle P, Maisonneuve P, Steg A: Decrease in mortality from benign prostatic hyperplasia: A major unheralded health triumph. J Urol 1996; 155:176–180.
21 Roehrborn CG, Boyle P, Bergner D, Gray T, Gittelman M, Shown T, Melman A, Bracken RB, de Vere White R, Taylor A, Wang D, Waldstreicher J: Serum prostate-specific antigen and prostate volume predict long-term changes in symptoms and flow rate: Results of a four-year, randomized trial comparing finasteride versus placebo. PLESS study group. Urology 1999;54:662–669.
22 Roehrborn CG, McConnell JD, Lieber M, Kaplan S, Geller J, Malek GH, Castellanos R, Coffield S, Saltzman B, Resnick M, Cook TJ, Waldstreicher J: Serum prostate-specific antigen concentration is a powerful predictor of acute urinary retention and need for surgery in men with clinical benign prostatic hyperplasia. PLESS study group. Urology 1999;53:473–480.
23 Michel MC, Mehlburger L, Bressel H-U, Schumacher H, Schäfers RF, Goepel M: Tamsulosin treatment of 19,365 patients with lower urinary tract symptoms: Does comorbidity alter tolerability? J Urol 1998;160:784–791.
24 Höfner K: Wirksamkeit und Sicherheit von Alfuzosin SR bei der BPH. Erfahrungen einer Anwendungsbeobachtung mit 11562 Patienten. Urologe B 1998;38:452–457.
25 Jardin A, Bensadoun H, Delauche-Cavallier MC, Attali P, The BPH-ALF Group: Alfuzosin for treatment of benign prostatic hypertrophy. Lancet 1991;337:1457–1461.
26 Michel MC, Bressel H-U, Goepel M, Rübben H: A 6-months large scale study into the safety of tamsulosin. Br J Clin Pharmacol 1999;48: 890P–891P.
27 Wasson JH, Reda DJ, Bruskewitz RC, Elinson J, Keller AM, Henderson WG: A comparison of transurethral surgery with watchful waiting for moderate symptoms of benign prostatic hyperplasia. New Engl J Med 1995;332:75–79.
28 McNeill SA, Daruwala PD, Mitchell IDC, Shearer MG, Hargreave TB: Sustained-release alfuzosin and trial without catheter after acute urinary retention: A prospective, placebo-controlled trial. BJU Int 1999;84:622–627.
29 Djavan B, Shariat S, Fakhari M, Ghawidel K, Seitz C, Partin AW, Roehrborn CG, Marberger M: Neoadjuvant and adjuvant alpha-blockade improves early results of high-energy transurethral microwave thermotherapy for lower urinary tract symptoms of benign prostatic hyperplasia: A randomized, prospective clinical trial. Urology 1999;53:251–259.
30 Michel MC, Schäfers RF, Goepel M: α-Blockers and lower urinary tract function: More than smooth muscle relaxation? BJU Int 2000; 86(suppl 2):23–30.
31 Knowlton KU, Michel MC, Itani M, Shubeita HE, Ishihara K, Brown JH, Chien KR: The α_{1A}-adrenergic receptor subtype mediates biochemical, molecular, and morphologic features of cultured myocardial cell hypertrophy. J Biol Chem 1993;268:15374–15380.
32 Yang M, Büscher R, Taguchi K, Grübbel B, Insel PA, Michel MC: Protein kinase C does not mediate phenylephrine-induced down-regulation of Madin-Darby canine kidney cell alpha-1B adrenoceptors. J Pharmacol Exp Ther 1998;286:36–43.
33 Xin X, Yang N, Eckhart AD, Faber JE: α_{1D}-Adrenergic receptors and mitogen-activated protein kinase mediate increased protein synthesis by arterial smooth muscle. Mol Pharmacol 1997;51:764–775.
34 Raff M: Cell suicide for beginners. Nature 1998;396:119–122.
35 Alexandrov A, Keffel S, Goepel M, Goepel M, Schulz R, Heusch G, Michel MC: Inhibition and enhancement of apoptosis by α_1-adrenoceptor stimulation. Br J Pharmacol 1999;128: 144P.
36 Kyprianou N, Litvak JP, Borkowski A, Jacobs SC: Induction of prostate apoptosis by doxazosin in benign prostatic hyperplasia. J Urol 1998;159:1810–1815.
37 Chon JK, Borkowski A, Partin AW, Isaacs JT, Jacobs SC, Kyprianou N: α_1-Adrenoceptor antagonists terazosin and doxazosin induce prostate apoptosis without affecting cell proliferation in patients with benign prostatic hyperplasia. J Urol 1999;161:2002–2008.
38 Cardillo M, Berchem G, Tarkington MA, Krajewski S, Krajewski M, Reed JC, Tehan T, Ortega L, Lage J, Gelmann EP: Resistance to apoptosis and up regulation of bcl-2 in benign prostatic hyperplasia after androgen deprivation. J Urol 1997;158:212–216.

European Urology

Eur Urol 2001;39(suppl 3):26–30

Lower Urinary Tract Symptoms Suggestive of Benign Prostatic Obstruction: What Are the Current Practice Patterns?

T.A. McNicholas

Department of Urology, Lister Hospital, Stevenage, UK

Key Words

Lower urinary tract symptoms · Benign prostatic obstruction · Medical therapy · Surgery · Primary care · Secondary care · Healthcare delivery

Abstract

Objective: The current clinical practice patterns for the management of LUTS suggestive of BPO in the US and in various European countries will be reviewed. ***Methods:*** Information was obtained from published scientific articles and IMS/GERS market analysis data. ***Results:*** Community-based surveys demonstrate that the prevalence of moderate to severe LUTS in elderly men is high and increases with age. The role of the GP in the initial management of LUTS is growing. In France, Italy and the UK, most patients with LUTS initially visit a GP. More and more patients in the US also first seek medical advice from a primary care physician or an internal medicine specialist. In Germany, both GPs and office-based urologists are involved in the initial management of LUTS. In Poland and Spain, office-based urologists initiate primary therapy for LUTS, although a trend towards involvement of GPs is also seen, especially in Poland. The shift in the initial management of LUTS from secondary to primary care accompanies a decreased incidence of surgery and a growing demand for medical therapy. Currently, there are considerable differences between the medical management of LUTS suggestive of BPO across Europe in real life practice. For example phytotherapy is particularly popular in countries such as Germany, France and Spain, whereas finasteride is more commonly used in Italy, Poland and the UK. α_1-Adrenoceptor antagonists are used in most of these countries as the primary treatment modality. The data furthermore suggest that the current management of patients is often more opinion- than evidence-based, which may at least partly be due to the fact that data on long-term effectiveness of treatment options in real life clinical practice are largely lacking. ***Conclusions:*** Due to the ageing and longevity of the population, the costs associated with the management of LUTS suggestive of BPO will rise in the future, whereas healthcare budgets will be relatively restricted. In order to improve cost-effective management of LUTS, more and better studies are needed in real life practice in primary care. These studies should not only be based on classical efficacy and safety data, but also on effectiveness of treatment in the long-term and the associated costs.

Introduction

Lower urinary tract symptoms (LUTS) suggestive of benign prostatic obstruction (BPO) is a common condition in the male population. Over the age of 40, the prevalence of LUTS suggestive of BPO is approximately 25%

KARGER

Fax + 41 61 306 12 34
E-Mail karger@karger.ch
www.karger.com

0302–2838/01/0399–0026$17.50/0

Accessible online at:
www.karger.com/journals/eur

T.A. McNicholas, MB.BS., FRCS, FEBU
Elm Tree House, Letchworth Lane
Letchworth, Herts SG6 3ND, UK
Tel. +44 1462 683814, Fax +44 1462 683815
E-Mail mcnic@globalnet.co.uk

[1, 2]. Due to the ageing and longevity of the population, the number of men suffering from LUTS is likely to increase in the future. Consequently, the costs associated with the management of LUTS will also grow. On the other hand, in developed countries the total population is slightly decreasing and therefore fewer younger people will be available to pay for the healthcare of an increased number of elderly. It is expected that in the future there will be deficits in healthcare budgets triggering more efficient use of resources. Therefore, more rational management of LUTS is needed, especially from a cost-effectiveness point of view.

Most evidence available today for the treatment of LUTS comes from randomised controlled trials (RCTs) performed in a secondary care setting. These trials are useful to retrieve information on 'short-term' efficacy (effect on LUTS and urinary flow) and safety of the different invasive and medical therapies. However, evidence from long-term studies is also needed to improve the cost-effective management of LUTS. More information about complications related to BPO and the incidence of switching to other medical therapy or surgery is needed, especially from real life practice (RLP) in primary care, since these are the major cost-drivers in the management of LUTS.

In order to translate the huge amount of scientific information on LUTS suggestive of BPO into meaningful recommendations on how to diagnose and manage LUTS in daily clinical practice, several organisations have developed practice guidelines. Among these, the Agency for Health Care Policy and Research (AHCPR/new name: Agency for Healthcare, Research and Quality (AHRQ)) [3] and the International Consultation on BPH [4] are the most comprehensive. However, limited information is currently available on how these guidelines are used in routine clinical practice. This review tries to summarise the current facts about the contemporary management of LUTS suggestive of BPO in the USA and in several European countries (i.e. France, Germany, Italy, Poland, Spain, UK).

Methods

In order to retrieve information about the prevalence and management of LUTS suggestive of BPO in the US and several European countries, a search was performed in Medline and Embase to obtain scientific articles describing the prevalence, healthcare delivery and/or treatment for LUTS for these countries. In addition, IMS/GERS market analysis data for medical therapy received from the pharmaceutical companies Boehringer Ingelheim and Yamanouchi Europe were taken into consideration.

Prevalence of LUTS

Although LUTS suggestive of BPO is a very common condition in elderly men, the reported prevalence differs between various studies, which can be due to the fact that different definitions of this condition are used [5]. Despite some country-specific differences, in general the prevalence of LUTS suggestive of BPO is estimated at 25% in men aged 40 years or over and increases up to about 40% in men over 65 years of age [1, 2, 6, 7]. These figures have been confirmed in recent, community-based studies. In Austria, the proportion of patients with an I-PSS >7 increased from 27.1% in men aged 50–59 years up to 36% in men aged 70–79 [8]. A community-based survey in more than 1,000 men aged 40 or older in Spain demonstrated a prevalence of moderate to severe LUTS of 25% [9]. In the UK, moderate to severe LUTS (I-PSS ≥8) occurred in 29–51% of a sample of 1,500 men aged 50 years or over, depending on the age group [10]. Overall, the prevalence of LUTS suggestive of BPO is high in the elderly male community and increases with age.

Healthcare Delivery in the US and throughout Europe

There appear to be differences in the healthcare delivery systems of the various countries discussed here with regard to the management of LUTS. In France, Italy and the UK most patients with LUTS initially visit their general practitioner (GP) [11–13]. A study in France in 1998 indicated that 64% of men initially sought medical advice with a GP for their bothersome LUTS, while 36% directly contacted a specialist (i.e. urologist or general surgeon) [11]. In some areas in the UK, the GP can refer the patient after the initial visit to a shared care clinic for reassurance of the diagnosis and for exclusion of prostate cancer. This type of clinic is supervised by a consultant urologist and managed by nursing staff who follows a tight diagnostic protocol. In case of suspicion of prostate cancer, the GP directly refers the patient to a urologist [13]. In the US, the importance of general medicine in LUTS management is growing and although in 37% of cases, patients initially visit a urologist, already 25% of patients with LUTS first seek medical advice from a primary care physician (PCP) and 24% consult an internal medicine specialist [14]. The fact that medical therapies are available as an alternative for surgery undoubtedly contributes to the growing role of general practice in the initial management of LUTS. General practitioners, office-based urologists and hospital-based urologists participate in the German healthcare system. Patients with bothersome LUTS can initially consult a GP or an office-based urologist, dependent on the patient's health insurance. Medical therapies are prescribed by both GPs and office-based urologists. GPs can refer the patient to an office-based or hospital-based urologist in case further diagnostic work-up is required or if the response to medical therapy is insufficient. In Germany, office-based urologists increasingly perform minimally invasive procedures (e.g. transurethral microwave therapy). When surgery or more invasive diagnostic tests need to be performed, patients will be referred to the hospital-based urologist [15]. In Poland and Spain, generally office-based urologists are involved in the initial management of LUTS, although especially in Poland GPs are playing an increasing role. A national survey in Spain among PCPs indicated that 95% of them directly refers patients with LUTS to a urologist, either without any investigation or after diagnostic evaluation or initial therapy [16].

It appears that GPs or Primary Care Groups (PCGs, in the UK) are actively managing patients with LUTS suggestive of BPO. Surveys in the UK and the US indicated that GPs or PCGs perform a digital rectal examination (DRE) and assess serum creatinine and prostate specific antigen (PSA) to diagnose LUTS and to exclude prostate cancer [13, 17, 18]. A French study in 1995 revealed that 89% of the participating GPs did a DRE, 75% investigated the presence of micturition disorders, but only 26% measured PSA [19].

Treatment Modalities for LUTS Suggestive of BPO

Surgical Therapy

In all countries, except the UK, the incidence of surgery is declining [20]. TURP is performed most frequently. In the UK, the incidence of prostatectomies has remained relatively stable, which is probably due to the fact that the number of practising urologists is limited and as a consequence, LUTS patients are put on a waiting list for a TURP [13]. In the US, TURP rates have declined about 50% during the early nineties, from more than 300,000/year in 1990 to approximately 150,000/year in 1995 [14, 21]. In Europe the application of surgery has also decreased, but to a lesser extent than in the US. In France, the incidence of prostatectomies was reduced by 36% and in Germany by 25% from 1990 to 1995 [20]. Although these data are already more than 5 years old, the consensus view is that this downward trend has continued. The decrease in surgery rates coincides with the availability of medical therapy for LUTS. Since 1995, more medical treatment options came on the market and therefore the incidence of surgery is expected to decrease further.

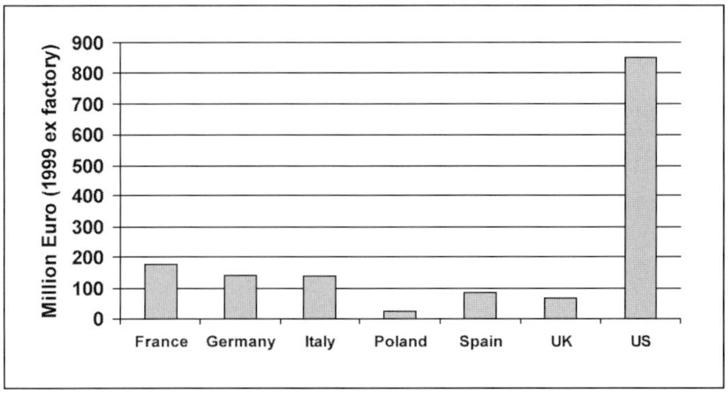

Fig. 1. Total cumulative 1999 ex factory sales (in Euro) for medical therapy in France, Germany, Italy, Poland, Spain, the UK and the US [22, 23].

The average cost/TURP differs considerably between various countries, with values of 2,000 Euro (UK), 3,000–3,500 Euro (France/Italy) and 7,500 Euro (US) [20]. This implies that the current average yearly costs for TURP are between 70 (UK) and 1,000 million Euro (US) [13, 14].

Medical Therapy

While the incidence of surgery is decreasing, the market for medical therapy is growing in both the US and Europe. This goes along with an increase in outpatient visits and a shift in the initial management of LUTS from secondary to primary care.

The total value of the market for medical therapy in 1999 was more than 800 million Euro in the US and around 150–180 million Euro in Germany, France and Italy (fig. 1) [22, 23]. The market for medical therapy in Poland and in the UK is much less. Compared to the other countries discussed here, the number of elderly people is lower in Poland (approximately 2 million). Thus also the number of males with LUTS is lower, which might explain the smaller market for medical therapy. In the UK, the number of elderly males is comparable to that living in France (approximately 4 million), so the difference is probably due to different prescribing patterns. Whereas many patients with mild or less bothersome LUTS in France might receive plant extracts, these patients may be on a watchful waiting regimen in the UK.

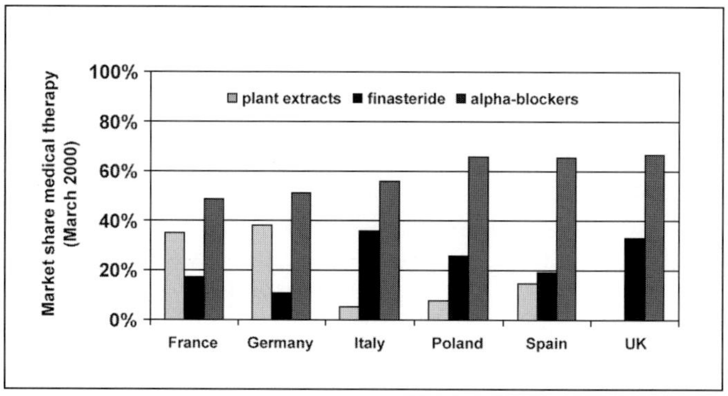

Fig. 2. Percentage market share (value March 2000) of phytotherapy, finasteride and α_1-adrenoceptor antagonists in France, Germany, Italy, Poland, Spain and the UK [22, 23].

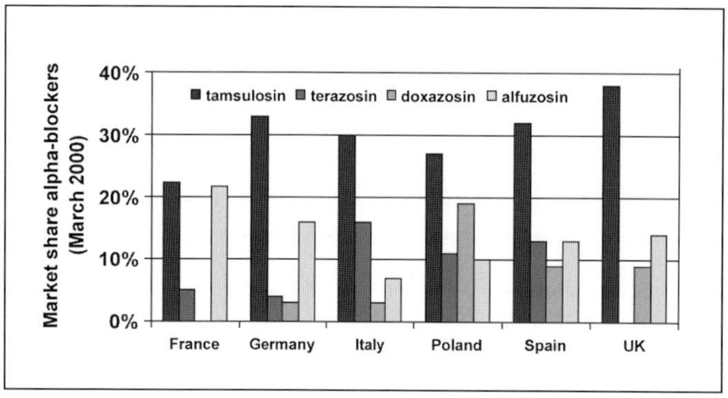

Fig. 3. Percentage market share (value March 2000) of α_1-adrenoceptor antagonists (tamsulosin, terazosin, doxazosin and alfuzosin) in France, Germany, Italy, Poland, Spain and the UK [22, 23].

Currently, there are considerable differences between the management of LUTS suggestive of BPO in RLP. In the US, α_1-adrenoceptor antagonists account for 82% of the total market and finasteride for only 18% (1999 sales). Figure 2 demonstrates that in Europe α_1-adrenoceptor antagonists are also used as a primary treatment modality (market shares between 50–67%). Phytotherapy is frequently used in France and Germany and to a lesser extent in Spain, with market shares of 35, 38 and 19% respectively (March 2000 sales). Finasteride is often prescribed in Italy (market share 36%), the UK (market share 33%) and Poland (market share 26%). Tamsulosin is the most frequently used α_1-adrenoceptor antagonist in all these countries (fig. 3). These data suggest that the current management of LUTS patients is very often based on the doctor's personal experience and patient preferences instead of on evidence. If prescribing information was purely based on scientific evidence from RCTs, then market shares for phytotherapy, finasteride and α_1-adrenoceptor antagonists would be similar across countries. This is not the case and might be due to cultural differences, e.g. plant extracts have always been available in Germany, France and Spain, and also because costs and reimbursements of various therapies differ between countries. Another factor may be that the currently available scientific evidence, which is mainly based on relatively short-term effects on classical efficacy (LUTS/flow) and safety data, is not sufficient for primary care physicians in daily life decision making. It is very important to know how many patients remain on initial therapy or how many medically treated patients eventually still proceed to surgery as these are the major contributors to the costs of the management of LUTS. This information is currently largely lacking. Bearing in mind the ageing and longevity of the population, the costs associated with the management of LUTS suggestive of BPO will rise in the future, whereas healthcare budgets will be relatively restricted. Therefore, cost-effective management of LUTS will be the major challenge for the future.

Conclusions

The prevalence of moderate to severe LUTS is high in elderly men and increases with age. In general, there appears to be a shift in the initial management of LUTS from secondary to primary care. This shift goes along with a declining incidence of surgery and a growing market for medical therapy. The medical management differs considerably between various countries, which implies that currently prescribing patterns are very often more opinion than evidence-based. This may at least partly be due to the fact that data on long-term effectiveness of treatment options in real life clinical practice are largely lacking. Since the costs associated with LUTS management will rise in the future due to the ageing and longevity of the population, it will be very important to improve cost-effective management of LUTS. Therefore, more and better studies are needed in real life practice in primary care, not only based on classical efficacy and safety factors, but also on the long-term effectiveness of treatment and the associated costs.

References

1 Garraway WM, Collins GN, Lee RJ: High prevalence of benign prostatic hypertrophy in the community. Lancet 1991;338:469–471.

2 Chute CG, Pander LA, Girman CJ, Oesterling JE, Guess HA, Jacobsen SJ, Lieber MM: The prevalence of prostatism: A population-based survey of urinary symptoms. J Urol 1993;150: 85–89.

3 McConnell JD, Barry MJ, Bruskewitz RC, et al: Clinical practice guideline for benign prostatic hyperplasia: Diagnosis and treatment. Rockeville, MD: Department of Health and Human Services, 1994. AHCPR publication no. 94-0582.

4 Denis L, McConnell J, Yoshida O, Khoury S, Abrams P, Barry M, Bartsch G, Cockett A, Corriere J, Dreikorn K, Gibbons R, Griffiths K, Hald T, Holtgrewe L, Jardin A, Koyanagi T, Mebust W, Murphy G, Roehrborn C, Smith P, and the members of the comittees; in Denis L, Griffiths K, Khoury S, Cockett ATK, McConnell J, Chatelain C, Murphy G, Yoshida O (eds): Proceedings of the 4th International Consultation on Benign Prostatic Hyperplasia (BPH), Paris, 1997 Jul 2–5. Plymouth Health Publication Ltd, 1998 pp 669–683.

5 Blanker MH, Groeneveld FPMJ, Prins A, Bernsen RMD, Bohnen AM, Bosch JLHR: Strong effects of definition and nonresponse bias on prevalence rates of clinical benign prostatic hyperplasia: The Krimpen study of male urogenital tract problems and general health status. BJU Int 2000;85:665–671.

6 Garraway WM, Russell EBAW, Lee RJ, Collins GN, McKelvie GB, Hehir M, Rogers ACN, Simpson RJ: Impact of previously unrecognised benign prostatic hyperplasia on the daily activities of middle-aged and elderly men. Br J Gen Pract 1993;43:318–321.

7 Bosch JLHR, Hop WJC, Kirkels WJ, Schröder FH: The International Prostate Symptom Score in a community-based sample of men between 55 and 74 years of age: Prevalence and correlation of symptoms with age, prostate volume, flow rate and residual urine volume. Br J Urol 1995;75:622–630.

8 Madersbacher S, Haidinger G, Temml C, Scmidbaucher CP, for the Prostate Study Group of the Austrian Society of Urology: Prevalence of lower urinary tract symptoms in Austria as assessed by an open survey of 2096 men. Eur Urol 1998;34:136–141.

9 Chicharro-Molero JA, Burgos-Rodriguez R, Sanchez-Cruz JJ, Del Rosal-Samaniego JM, Rodero-Carcia P, Rodriguez-Vallejo JM: Prevalence of benign prostatic hyperplasia in Spanish men 40 years old or older. J Urol 1998;159: 878–882.

10 Trueman P, Hood SC, Nayak USL, Mrazek MF: Prevalence of lower urinary tract symptoms and self-reported diagnosed 'benign prostatic hyperplasia', and their effect on quality of life in a community-based survey of men in the UK. BJU International 1999;83:410–415.

11 Lukacs B: Management of symptomatic BPH in France: Who is treated and how? Eur Urol 1999;36(suppl 3):14–20.

12 Tubaro A, Montanari E: Management of symptomatic BPH in Italy: Who is treated and how? Eur Urol 1999;36(suppl 3):28–32.

13 McNicholas TA: Management of symptomatic BPH in the UK: Who is treated and how? Eur Urol 1999;36(suppl 3):33–39.

14 Bruskewitz R: Management of symptomatic BPH in the US: Who is treated and how? Eur Urol 1999;36(suppl 3):7–13.

15 Berges RR, Pientka L: Management of symptomatic BPH in Germany: Who is treated and how? Eur Urol 1999;36(suppl 3):21–27.

16 Jimenez Cruz JF, Rodriguez Vallejo JM, Conejero J, Resel L, Rioja LA, Vela Navarette R, Vicente J: Primary care physicians and prostatic disease. National survey. Members of the Spanish Council of Prostatic Health. Actas Urol Esp 1996;20:624–629.

17 Fawzy A, Fontenot C, Guthrie R, Baudier MM: Practice patterns among primary care physicians in benign prostatic hyperplasia and prostate cancer. Fam Med 1997;29:321–325.

18 McNaughton Collins M, Barry MJ, Lin B, Roberts RG, Oesterling JE, Fowler FJ: Diagnosis and treatment of benign prostatic hyperplasia. Practice patterns of primary care physicians. J Gen Intern Med 1997;12:224–229.

19 Coeurdacier P, Staerman F, Thoquenne G, Cipolla B, Guillé F, Lobel B: Le médecin généraliste face aux troubles mictionnels de l'homme de plus de 50 ans. 250 médecins interrogés en Bretagne. Prog Urol 1996;6:52–59.

20 Holtgrewe HL, Bay-Nielsen H, Carlsson P, Coast J, Echtle D, Fitzpatrick F, Garcia Perez M, Lanson Y, Melchior H, Standaert B, Vallancien G: The economics of the management of lower urinary tract symptoms and benign prostatic hyperplasia; in Denis L, Griffiths K, Khoury S, Cockett ATK, McConnell J, Chatelain C, Murphy G, Yoshida O (eds): Proceedings of the 4th International Consultation on Benign Prostatic Hyperplasia (BPH). Plymouth, Plymbridge Distributors, 1998, pp 61–81.

21 Baine WB, Yu W, Summe JP, Weis KA: Epidemiologic trends in the evaluation and treatment of lower urinary tract symptoms in elderly male Medicare patients from 1991 to 1995. J Urol 1998;160:816–820.

22 IMS market analysis data.

23 GERS (Groupement pour l'élaboration et la realisation de statistiques) market analysis data.

European Urology

Eur Urol 2001;39(suppl 3):31–36

Lower Urinary Tract Symptoms Suggestive of Benign Prostatic Obstruction – Triumph: Design and Implementation

Christopher R. Chapple
on behalf of the Pan-European Expert Panel (Appendix 1)

Department of Urology, Royal Hallamshire Hospital, Sheffield, UK

Key Words
Lower urinary tract symptoms · Benign prostatic obstruction · Medical therapy · Cost-effectiveness · Treatment failure · Long-term · Triumph

Abstract
Lower urinary tract symptoms (LUTS) suggestive of benign prostatic obstruction (BPO) are likely to become an increasing burden for health care budgets in the future due to the high prevalence of this condition in the elderly and the ageing of the population. Data on the cost-effectiveness of the available treatment options in order to promote rational management will therefore be crucial. As this information is currently largely lacking, the European Association of Urology (EAU) has endorsed the formation of a Pan-European Expert Panel that has developed the Triumph (TransEuropean Research Into the Use of Management Policies for LUTS suggestive of BPH in Primary Healthcare) project. The Triumph project will evaluate how LUTS suggestive of BPO is currently managed in real life practice in initially 6 European countries (France, Germany, Italy, Poland, Spain and the UK) and how this condition progresses over time in relation to an initial treatment choice. In other words, how many patients remain on their initial therapy, how many switch to another therapy (including surgery) and within which time frame and how many develop serious complications related to BPO such as acute urinary retention. The clinical data will be retrieved from continuous analysis of large computer-based patient files such as the General Practice Research Database (GPRD) in the UK and the Integrated Primary Care Information (IPCI) database in The Netherlands. Furthermore, a cross-sectional, observational survey will gather similar data in a prospective fashion for at least 1 year from approximately 13,000 patients managed by more than 1,000 primary care physicians in all 6 countries. Both newly diagnosed (around 7,500) and existing (around 5,500) LUTS patients will be enrolled. For the existing patients in whom the diagnosis was made in the past (from January 1997 onwards), the relevant retrospective data (up to 3.5 years) on disease progression will also be collected. Finally, the costs associated with these treatments will be investigated by the development of a national costing database for each participating country that will detail costs related to visits, investigations, prescriptions, surgical interventions, etc. The last patient is anticipated to come out of the initial prospective survey by the end of 2002/beginning of 2003 and the results will hopefully contribute to improved cost-effective management of LUTS suggestive of BPO in the future.

KARGER
Fax + 41 61 306 12 34
E-Mail karger@karger.ch
www.karger.com

0302–2838/01/0399–0031$17.50/0

Accessible online at:
www.karger.com/journals/eur

C.R. Chapple
Department of Urology, Royal Hallamshire Hospital
Glossop Road
Sheffield S10 2JF (UK)
Tel. +44 114 271 3047, Fax +44 114 279 7841, E-Mail c.r.chapple@sheffield.ac.uk

Introduction

Lower urinary tract symptoms (LUTS) suggestive of benign prostatic obstruction (BPO), previously referred to as symptomatic benign prostatic hyperplasia (BPH), is a common condition in elderly men. It occurs in 25% of men aged 40 years and over and its prevalence increases with age [1].

In the 1980s, LUTS suggestive of BPO was predominantly managed in secondary care with two options available: surgery for patients with absolute indications (e.g. acute urinary retention (AUR), haematuria, recurrent urinary tract infections (UTIs) or bladder stones) or moderate to severe LUTS and no medication with regular follow-up (watchful waiting) for those with mild LUTS. In the last decade of the previous millennium, the management of this condition however changed enormously, predominantly due to the introduction of effective and well tolerated medical treatment options such as finasteride and several α_1-adrenoceptor antagonists (alfuzosin, doxazosin, tamsulosin and terazosin). This resulted in a substantial decline in the number of transurethral resections of the prostate (TURPs) performed, an increase in the usage of medical therapies and a shift in the treatment of this condition from a secondary care to a primary care setting [2].

Due to the ageing of the population in Europe (fig. 1), the number of men who will suffer from and will seek medical advice for LUTS is expected to increase dramatically in the next 25 years. Whereas currently approximately 15% of the population is aged 65 years or over, this is anticipated to increase to up to 25% in 2025. Furthermore, these patients will live longer while expecting a maintained quality of life. Therefore, the expenditure for medical therapies will also increase tremendously. It is however not very realistic to expect a similar increase in health care budgets as these are already becoming more and more restricted. Consequently, for the future rational management of LUTS suggestive of BPO based on the available scientific evidence, especially from a cost-effectiveness point of view, will become more and more crucial.

It is clear that accurate and robust cost-effectiveness data on the treatment of LUTS are very limited [3]. Therefore, the EAU has endorsed a group of experts in the field of urology, primary care, pharmaco-epidemiology and pharmaco-economics to develop a programme that should provide insight into this issue. This Pan-European Expert Panel designed the Triumph project, the abbreviation for "TransEuropean Research Into the Use of Management Policies for LUTS suggestive of BPH in Primary Healthcare". It can be regarded as one of the largest current research projects in LUTS suggestive of BPO.

Table 1. Major objectives of the Triumph project

1	How is LUTS suggestive of BPO currently managed in several European countries?
2	What are the costs associated with the current management approaches?
3	How does LUTS suggestive of BPO progress: which complications due to BPO develop, how frequently and within which time frame and how many patients will finally proceed to surgery?
4	What is the difference between currently applied treatment approaches for LUTS suggestive of BPO with regard to disease progression and costs?
5	Can relevant improvements in cost-effective delivery of health care for LUTS suggestive of BPO be realised by applying the most appropriate management approach?

Objectives

Treatment failure and subsequent cascade management are the major cost-drivers in LUTS [3]. The Triumph project will therefore not only assess the effect of initial treatment options on classical efficacy parameters such as relief of symptoms (reduction in International Prostate Symptom Score (I-PSS)) and improvement in quality of life (IPSS-QoL), but it will also focus on both treatment failure and disease progression. This is evaluated by following individual patients over time and documenting whether patients remain on their initial treatment or switch to other treatment; the possibilities being no medication but follow-up (watchful waiting), medical therapy or referral to secondary care for surgery. Disease progression will be monitored by documenting the development of complications related to BPO such as AUR, recurrent UTIs, haematuria, bladder stones or renal dysfunction. In addition to gathering clinical data on the long-term effectiveness and efficacy of initial treatment approaches, costs will be investigated (see table 1).

Design

The Triumph project will initially run in 6 countries in Europe: France, Germany, Italy, Poland, Spain and the United Kingdom (UK). The project consists of several steps that are briefly described below.

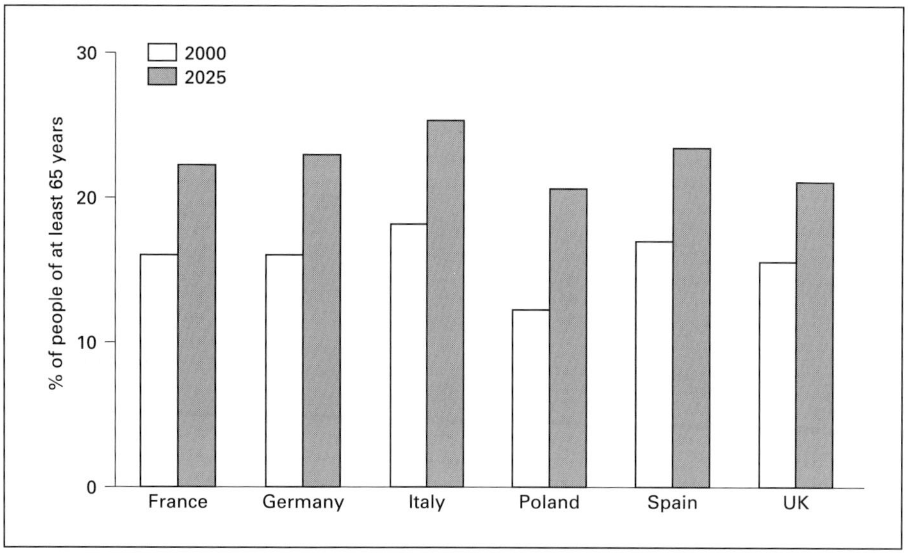

Fig. 1. Anticipated growth of the elderly population in several European countries (U.S. Census Bureau, <http://www.census.gov>; 21-03-2000).

Step 1: Analysis of Primary Care Databases

Patient medical records contain numerous data on individual patients who are followed up. They can therefore be a valuable first tool for retrieving information on the effectiveness of different applied treatment options in real life practice, e.g. for LUTS suggestive of BPO. Unfortunately, most medical records are at present only paper-based and can therefore only with difficulty be used for research purposes (for instance by classical chart review). Classical chart review based on a pre-defined questionnaire is both time- and manpower-consuming and is consequently a very costly process. In some countries such as the UK, The Netherlands, Italy and France computer-based systems have been increasingly used for research purposes. The electronic patient files that are consulted as part of the Triumph project are briefly reviewed below.

In the UK, the General Practice Research Database (GPRD) is currently owned and quality-controlled under the supervision of the UK Medicines Control Agency (MCA) [4]. It is Europe's largest computerised database of anonymised longitudinal patient medical records. Currently it contains the records of approximately 4.6 million people registered with around 450 general practices (each comprising 3 or more physicians), i.e. around 8% of the population in England and Wales. Not surprisingly therefore, the UK Office of National Statistics (ONS) produces a regular publication of key health statistics from the GPRD. The electronic records contain coded information on basic patient demographics, diagnoses, investigations, prescriptions and hospital referrals, i.e. observations deemed relevant for patient care at the moment of entrance into the system. The GPRD can therefore for instance be used to calculate how many patients with LUTS were diagnosed within a particular time frame, their prescription pattern over time and whether or not they were admitted to hospital for prostatic surgery or underwent catheterisation (a proxy for acute urinary retention). Currently, the database covers around 60,000 patients with LUTS or a diagnosis of BPH managed from 1992 onwards in primary care. As part of the Triumph project, the University of Surrey in the UK will perform continuous updates and analyses of this subset of patients over the coming years to assess the long-term effectiveness of initial LUTS treatment options in primary care. For more detailed information and preliminary results, refer to the paper by Farmer and colleagues in this supplement [5].

In the Netherlands, the Erasmus University in Rotterdam runs a similar database to the GPRD, the Integrated Primary Care Information (IPCI) database [6]. This project was initiated in 1992 and currently 150 GPs managing 485,000 patients (about 3% of the total Dutch population) are contributing to this database by solely using electronic patient files. The files include information on patient characteristics, prescriptions, indications for therapy, physical findings, referrals, etc. Similar analyses will be performed on this database as for the GPRD.

Step 2: Prospective, Observational Survey

In addition to the use of database material, a prospective, cross-sectional, observational (i.e. non-interventional) survey will be conducted in all 6 countries. A total of

Table 2. Number of patients planned to be included in the prospective, observational Triumph survey

	Existing	New	ALL
France	1,100	1,100	2,200
Germany	1,080	1,080	2,160
Italy	1,100	1,100	2,200
Poland	1,100	1,100	2,200
Spain	1,100	1,100	2,200
UK	0*	2,000	2,000
Total	5,480	7,480	~13,000**

* Continuous update GPRD; ** >70,000 patients including GPRD.

13,000 men with LUTS will be enrolled across these countries (see table 2). This will include both 'existing' patients diagnosed with LUTS suggestive of BPO from 1 January 1997 onwards (n = 5,480) and 'newly diagnosed' patients (n = 7,480). As the UK (GPRD) will provide information on over 60,000 patients with LUTS/BPH followed up since 1992, only newly diagnosed patients will be included in the prospective survey in this country.

Both existing and newly diagnosed patients will be prospectively followed for at least 1 year. During this period, baseline characteristics (e.g. age, co-morbidity, symptom severity and disease-specific quality of life (I-PSS questionnaire)), treatment choice and major events related to treatment failure/disease progression such as switch to other therapy (including prostatic surgery) or serious complications related to BPO such as AUR will be collected. For the existing patients, the physicians also provide retrospective data referring back to the time of diagnosis and documenting initial treatment, therapy switches and development of BPO complications based on the patient medical record and/or patient interview (see table 3). The Triumph project will therefore collect up to 4.5-year data on disease progression: up to 3.5 years retrospectively for the existing patients and 1 year prospectively for the existing and newly diagnosed patients. It is hoped that ongoing prospective review of these patients for longer periods of time will be continued in the future.

In order to achieve these aims the Triumph project will recruit more than 1,000 primary care physicians across the initial 6 countries who will also be asked to document therapeutic interventions in the patients which occur if and when they are treated in a secondary care setting. In France and the UK, general practitioners (GPs) have become more and more heavily involved in the initial treatment of LUTS and tend only to refer patients to (hospital-based) urologists for confirmation of diagnosis in equivocal cases or in the context of unsatisfactory response to initial therapy. In Poland and Spain office-based urologists act as primary care physicians and are to a large extent responsible for both the diagnostic work up and the initial management of LUTS patients. Patients are referred to hospital only in situations where prostatic surgery seems to be necessary. Although in Italy, GPs do not traditionally supervise the treatment of patients presenting with LUTS, only drug prescriptions from GPs are reimbursed and therefore the GPs, who often also have a lifelong relationship with the patient, are central to the clinical management of patients in Italy. For these reasons, GPs have been selected as the responsible primary care physicians in the Triumph project for France, Italy and the UK and office-based urologists for Poland and Spain. In contrast in Germany, both GPs and office-based urologists can actively manage LUTS patients and therefore both groups will participate in the Triumph project (see table 4) [7]. In the southern part of the Netherlands, 14 GP practices will also document the usual care management of around 450 existing and newly diagnosed patients with LUTS (I-PSS ≥ 8) on the data collection forms specifically designed for the Triumph survey.

Step 3: Health-Economical Aspects

An important question remains as to how costs will be documented and which particular health-economic data will be obtained from the Triumph project. This aspect of the project will be co-ordinated by health-economists working at the Erasmus University in Rotterdam. They will develop a national costing database for each of the participating countries based on hospital information systems, physician interviews, etc. The costing database will contain cost estimates of visits, investigations, prescriptions and surgical interventions. The clinical data obtained in the prospective, observational survey can then be linked to the relevant cost estimates in the national costing databases to perform the cost-effectiveness analysis. A health-economics model will furthermore be constructed that will initially be based on the data from the GRPD and will be refined using the data from the prospective, observational survey. The model will be rendered country-specific by including more detailed information on national costs and health care delivery information. Finally, they will develop and validate disease states based on the I-PSS questionnaire that will enable quality-adjusted life years (QALYs) calculation based on

Table 3. Major events documented in the prospective, observational Triumph survey

		Inclusion V0		Follow-up V1, V2, V..	Final VF
		existing	new		
DCF	Selection criteria	√	√		
	Demographic details	√	√		
	Co-morbidity	√	√	√	√
	Co-medication	√	√	√	√
	Examination	√	√	√	√
	Switch to other LUTS therapy	√		√	√
	Serious LUTS complications	√		√	√
	Initial treatment approach	√	√		
	Referral to secondary care	√	√	√	√
	Decision of secondary care			√	√
Patient questionnaire	I-PSS/QoL	√	√	√	√
	Patient satisfaction	√		√	√

DCF = Data collection form; V0 = visit 0/initial visit, V1 = first follow-up visit, VF = final visit, 1-year following inclusion in case no follow-up visit took place.

the I-PSS data collected in the prospective, observational survey. For more information on health economics in general and in relation to the Triumph project and preliminary results, refer to the paper by Van Busschbach and Rutten [8].

Table 4. Number and type of physicians participating in the prospective, observational Triumph survey

Country	Type of physician	Number
France	GPs	220
Germany	GPs	120
	Office-based urologists	40
Italy	GPs	220
Poland	Office-based urologists	75
Spain	Office-based urologists	75
UK	GPs	400–500
Total		1,150–1,250

Implementation and Communication

The protocol and data collection form of the prospective, cross-sectional, observational survey were finalised in the first-second quarter of 2000. In those countries where ethical committee (EC) approval was required (France, Germany, Spain and the UK), submission took place in the second quarter of 2000. Several state-specific or local EC approvals have been obtained in the meanwhile in most countries and this is ongoing for other states/local ECs. In the UK, Multiple Research EC (MREC) approval has also been granted and Local Research EC (LREC) submission and approval is continuing at a local level.

Mailings have been sent out to primary care physicians in five countries (Germany, Italy, Poland, Spain and the UK) during the third and fourth quarters of 2000 to canvass their interest in participating in this important research project. A national network of GPs called Euraxi will run the survey in France. So far (beginning November 2000), almost 550 physicians have received all survey-related materials and the first 232 patients (151 existing and 81 newly diagnosed) have already been enrolled.

Progress of the project will be communicated at national and international congresses and on the web site http://www.mens-care.org. During the course of the project, yearly interim analyses will be performed and supervised by the Pan-European Expert Panel. The last patient will come out of the prospective survey by the end of 2002/beginning of 2003. Final analysis of the first phase of this project will therefore be available in the first half of 2003.

Conclusion

The results of the Triumph project will for the first time provide insight into the effect of different treatment options on health outcomes which are responsible for driving costs in the management of LUTS suggestive of BPO in real life practice. Hopefully, the Triumph project will also provide the basis and direction for us to improve the cost-effective management of an ageing and increasing population of patients with LUTS suggestive of BPO in the future.

Acknowledgement

The Triumph survey is sponsored by an unconditional educational grant from Yamanouchi Europe B.V. Furthermore, the Pan-European Expert Panel wants to express their gratitude to Ismar Healthcare N.V. for their support in developing, implementing and overviewing the project management of the survey.

Appendix 1

Members of the Pan-European Expert Panel

Name	City	Country	Discipline
W. Artibani	Verona	Italy	Urology
B. Begaud	Bordeaux	France	Pharmaco-epidemiology
R. Berges	Herne	Germany	Urology
A. Borkowski	Warsaw	Poland	Urology
C.R. Chapple*	Sheffield	UK	Urology
P. Dobronski	Warsaw	Poland	Urology
R.D.T. Farmer	Guildford	UK	Pharmaco-epidemiology
F. Jiménez Cruz	Valencia	Spain	Urology
U. Jonas	Hannover	Germany	Urology
K. MacRae	London	UK	Biostatistics
L. Pientka	Bochum	Germany	Geriatrics
F.F.H. Rutten	Rotterdam	The Netherlands	Pharmaco-economics
C.P. van Schayck	Maastricht	The Netherlands	Primary care medicine
M.J. Speakman	Taunton	UK	Urology
P. Teillac	Paris	France	Urology
A. Tubaro	L'aquila	Italy	Urology
G. Vallancien	Paris	France	Urology
R. Vela Navarrete	Madrid	Spain	Urology

* Chairman.

References

1 Garraway WM, Russell EBAW, Lee RJ, Collins GN, McKelvie GB, Hehir M, Rogers ACN, Simpson RJ: Impact of previously unrecognized benign prostatic hyperplasia on the daily activities of middle-aged and elderly men. Br J Gen Pract 1993;43:318–321.
2 Chapple CR: Introduction and concluding remarks. Eur Urol 1999;36(suppl 3):1–6.
3 Speakman MJ: Who should be treated and how? Evidence-based medicine on symptomatic BPH. Eur Urol 1999;36(suppl 3):40–51.
4 http://www.gprd.com
5 Logie JW, Clifford GM, Farmer RDT, Meesen BPW: Lower urinary tract symptoms suggestive of benign prostatic obstruction. Triumph: the role of general practice databases. Eur Urol 2001;39(suppl 3):42–47.
6 http://www.ipci.nl
7 McNicholas TA: Lower urinary tract symptoms suggestive of benign prostatic obstruction. What are the current practice patterns? Eur Urol 2001;39(suppl 3):26–30.
8 McDonnell J, Van Busschbach JJV, Kok E, van Exel J, Stolk E, Koopmanschap M, Rutten FFH: Lower urinary tract symptoms suggestive of benign prostatic obstruction. Triumph: health-economical analysis. Eur Urol 2001;39(suppl 3):37–41.

European Urology

Eur Urol 2001;39(suppl 3):37–41

Lower Urinary Tract Symptoms Suggestive of Benign Prostatic Obstruction – Triumph: Health-Economical Analysis

Joseph McDonnell Jan J.V. Busschbach Esther Kok Job van Exel Elly Stolk Marc Koopmanschap Frans F.H. Rutten

Institute for Medical Technology Assessment, Erasmus University, Rotterdam, The Netherlands

Key Words

Lower urinary tract symptoms · Benign prostatic obstruction · Cost-effectiveness · Health-economics · QALY · Economic model

Abstract

Given the ageing of western populations, the cost burden associated with the treatment of LUTS suggestive of BPO will increase substantially over the next few decades. Therefore, from the economic perspective, the primary objective of the Triumph project is the assessment of the cost-effectiveness of treatment options for lower urinary tract symptoms (LUTS) suggestive of benign prostatic obstruction (BPO), formerly referred to as symptomtic benign prostatic hyperplasia (BPH), in medical practice in initially six European countries. All modalities of LUTS treatment used in these countries will be considered. The effectiveness and costs associated with these treatments will be assessed in each country. Data will be gathered from observed medical practice rather than in the setting of a trial. Country-specific aspects will be studied and the outcome of country-specific policies can be predicted. Patient quality of life will also be measured using the I-PSS score as a basis. A number of treatment scenarios will be assessed in terms of both their costs and long-term effects, using a computer simulation. These economic analyses will provide greatly improved insight into the most cost-effective treatments for LUTS suggestive of BPO.

Introduction

From the economic perspective, the primary objective of the Triumph survey is the assessment of the cost-effectiveness of treatment options for lower urinary tract symptoms (LUTS) suggestive of benign prostatic obstruction (BPO), formerly referred to as symptomtic benign prostatic hyperplasia (BPH), in medical practice. For this purpose, all modalities of LUTS treatment used in the six initial survey countries (France, Germany, Italy, Poland, Spain and the UK) will be considered. Relevant treatment scenarios will be assessed in terms of both their costs and long-term effects, i.e. the possibility of switching between treatment options, eventual progression to prostatic surgery and eventual development of serious complications related to BPO such as acute urinary retention (AUR). As we are interested in cost effectiveness in daily practice rather than cost efficacy as measured in a controlled trial situation, the source of information for this survey is observed medical practice. For this reason, data collection must be done in such a way that the impact of the research

KARGER

Fax + 41 61 306 12 34
E-Mail karger@karger.ch
www.karger.com

0302–2838/01/0399–0037$17.50/0

Accessible online at:
www.karger.com/journals/eur

Joseph McDonnell
Institute for Medical Technology Assessment, Erasmus University
PO Box 1738
NL–3000 DR Rotterdam (The Netherlands)
Tel. +31 10 408 8571, Fax +31 10 408 9092, E-Mail mcdonnell@bmg.eur.nl

on observed practice is minimal. Because the economic analysis will be based on international data, country-specific aspects can be studied and the outcome of country-specific policies can be predicted. The following article gives an introduction into economic evaluation and its operationalisation in urology within the Triumph project.

Economic Evaluation

Economic evaluation is becoming increasingly important in developing health policy. Until fairly recently, the application of new interventions in health care were determined by rules of safety and efficacy. However the growth in health care expenditure and the ageing of the population has forced governments all over the world to incorporate economic considerations in their health care policy. For this reason, many countries now require estimates of the economic impact of new medication (relative to the impact of health) before they consider reimbursement.

Economic evaluation is usually associated with the calculation of the total costs of an intervention, for example, the total costs of prostate surgery. However, such straight forward calculations are of limited value if one fails to take the effects of the intervention on health into account. Thus in order to get a meaningful estimation of the cost-effectiveness of an intervention it is necessary to compare the costs in relation with the effects. Consequently, much research effort in economic evaluation is put into the measurement of the effects of health care on the health status of the patients.

Naturalistic versus Randomised Controlled Trials

Randomised controlled trials (RCTs) are the basis for modern ‘evidence-based medicine’. They are considered by many to be the gold standard in proving causality and demonstrating efficacy in clinical research. However, this efficacy refers only to how well an intervention or drug works in an ‘ideal’ situation such as a randomised, double-blind, phase III trial. In the normal clinical situation, such ideal situations are rarely, if ever, encountered. For example, typical patients are not selected using well-defined in- and exclusion criteria and, in practice, patients may switch to alternative therapies if the initial therapy does not seem to be effective. There are other points of substantial difference. In normal practice, compliance is not strictly monitored, and the costs of prescription of drugs are often high within a trial and much lower in practice. In other words, the efficacy of trial results and the cost implications resulting from a trial cannot readily be extrapolated to estimate cost-effectiveness in everyday practice.

The branch of science which attempts to determine the effectiveness of a treatment is called ‘outcome research’ and typically tries to combine trial data with observational studies; it therefore has a strong epidemiological component. Health economics is closely linked to outcome research in that health economics attempts to estimate both the costs and effects of a drug or other intervention in real life. As stated above, trial data is of limited value for the estimation of the real costs. Given that the Triumph survey is a (large-scale) real life (naturalistic) prospective survey, it offers a unique opportunity to provide insight into the real economics behind the management of LUTS. Indeed, this survey can be regarded as one of the largest naturalistic studies ever performed in Europe, with data being collected on the treatments, use of resources and symptomatology for approximately 13,000 patients.

A naturalistic study has an entirely different design to that of a RCT. Typically, no control group exists or is present only in the form of a ‘quasi control group’; such groups may exist in a different location (e.g. in a different country or province) or at another time (before and after the introduction of a new intervention). In a RCT, randomisation is used to minimise differences between patient groups. This is not possible in a naturalistic study design. Differences in the clinical characteristics of the groups must therefore be taken into account in the analysis. The design used in such studies often closely resembles those used in economic and sociological research. In these sciences, it is rarely possible to test hypotheses in a randomised setting, and alternative methodologies have been developed. These are typically based on statistical modelling and attempt to control for observed differences between groups. For example, in an economic study, when testing the effect of a given intervention on unemployment between countries, one might wish to adjust the measurements of unemployment using differences in gross national product, as gross national product may heavily confound any analysis on the level of unemployment in a given country.

It should be stressed that naturalistic study designs should not be seen as substitutes for RCTs. RCTs are the only research design that can ‘determine’ causality in an unambivalent fashion. Naturalistic designs are complementary in that they can indicate if treatment effects are likely to occur in real practice.

Two kinds of databases will be available for the Triumph survey, one a historical, the other a prospectively collected database in each of the six countries. The historical databases are the General Practice Research Database (GPRD) in the UK and the Integrated Primary Care Information (IPCI database) in the Netherlands. The GPRD is a unique database containing anonymous medical records from around 450 primary care practices serving about 4.2 million people in the UK. This database can provide information on a number of important aspects of treatment for LUTS suggestive of BPO, such as the type and effect of initial treatment, the time to change in therapy (and the reason for that change) and on time to surgery. However, since the data was not collected with the needs of the Triumph survey in mind, some important and relevant aspects on patient characteristics, particularly at baseline, are unavailable. Moreover, it does not contain a standardised BPH symptom score, making it difficult to obtain a detailed picture of the natural history of the disease. Costs and effects will be influenced not only by type of treatment but also by patient characteristics and severity of illness, both at baseline and during follow-up. Accordingly, the prospective data set will include data on patient characteristics and symptomatology both at baseline and during follow-up. This dataset will allow us to produce unbiased estimates of cost effectiveness.

Costs

Health care budgets are limited and the cost of interventions play an important role in health policy decisions. The Triumph project will therefore investigate the costs associated with the treatment options for LUTS suggestive of BPO. In determining these costs, we use a 'societal' perspective. This means two things. First, in calculating the costs of an intervention, we do not generally investigate tariffs and actual expenditures, but rather measure the resource use related with the specific intervention. Resources include time, medication (and other material costs), occupation of a hospital bed (i.e. capital costs), and so on. The societal perspective also means that we estimate not only the costs incurred within the health care sector itself, but the costs incurred by the patient or others in society, in so far as they are related with the intervention. For example, this view includes not only the time a health professional invests in an intervention (and the associated costs), but also the productivity time lost by the patient (and/or family members). For all costs such as visits to general practitioners or urologists, hospitalisation, LUTS medication, prostatic surgery, serious complications related to BPO such as AUR, etc. average estimates will be made for each of the participating countries.

It is inevitable that treatment patterns (surgical interventions, diagnostic procedures, laboratory tests and drug use) and resource costs (referral to specialists) will differ from country to country. Consequently, cost information will be collected in each country and a country-specific cost profile for each LUTS treatment will be produced.

Some cost information will be found in national registries or existing national cost studies, but for a number of more complex procedures the necessary information will need to be collected by means of an in-depth on-site cost investigation. As availability and usefulness of information from local accounting departments in hospitals and other sources will differ, the method of data collection will differ across countries. Given this variation in circumstances, analysing the data will also be a major research effort and support of local experts will be required not only in the collection of data but also in deriving conclusions from the analysis.

Health Effects

In clinical research, effects measured are often physiological parameters such as blood pressure and infection counts. However, this strategy may be of limited value when rather different interventions are compared. In the Triumph survey, we will therefore evaluate the long-term effectiveness of initial treatment options (for primary care physicians these will be predominantly watchful waiting, medical therapy or referral to secondary care). This implies that we will focus on disease progression with each initial therapy determined by the switch to other therapy (including prostatic surgery) and the development of serious complications related to BPO. The aspect of time is usually not incorporated in the analyses. Clearly, the time a patient has to endure the symptoms of a disease is of major importance, particularly to the patient. For this reason, epidemiologists and health economists have a long tradition of developing outcome measures which represent health status over time. In both sciences, the state of the art is the outcome measure 'quality adjusted life years' (QALYs).

In a QALY-analysis, life years of a patient are 'corrected' for the value of quality of life. Usually, the value for the quality of life is expressed as a value with a range from 0 to 1. In such analysis 0 stands for a quality of life equal to the value of death and 1 for a value of quality of life equal to normal health. Usually these values are determined with quality of life questionnaires, such as the EuroQol EQ-5D and the Health Utility Index (HUI), which have been specially designed and validated. However, it is unlikely that these generic quality of life questionnaires will be sufficiently sensitive for the effects of LUTS and its treatment, if for no other reason that questionnaires do not ask about LUTS-related problems such as micturition problems. For this reason the Triumph project has conducted a validation project, in which QALYs are derived from the well-known International Prostate Symptom Score (I-PSS).

The I-PSS is a 7-item questionnaire, which allows the patient to answer the questions on a 6-point scale. This means that it is theoretically possible to classify a patient into one of 279,936 (6^7) health states. The I-PSS can be made applicable for use in economic evaluation by attributing quality of life weights to each of these health states. This is done by converting the health states of the I-PSS into quality of life values using the time trade of interview technique.

The number of possible health states is too high for these methods to be immediately applicable. Therefore, it is necessary that the number of health states be reduced. To this end, we performed a factor analysis. This analysis revealed two factors, which are equivalent to the classical distinction 'irritative' (or 'filling') and 'obstructive' (or 'voiding') factors. These factors have also been found in other research [1]. The obstructive factor reflects the physical problems with urinating, while the irritative factor describes the bothersomeness a patient experiences due to the frequency and urgency of urinating. To further reduce the number of health states, we reduced the number of levels associated with each factor to three, namely seldom/never (1), about half the time or sometimes (2) and almost always (3). Using these levels, there are just 9 (3*3) unique health states for valuation.

The I-PSS can then be valued in the same way as QALY-instruments such as the EuroQol and the HUI using the 'time trade-off' procedure. Respondents were presented with a series of descriptions of health states relating to voiding problems. For each state, they were asked to imagine that their own health state was identical to that state. They were then asked how many years (if any) they would be willing to sacrifice in return for full health. For a description of this method see Drummond et al. [2] or Stolk et al. [3] for examples in the field of urology. To examine whether the method provides valid results, we first tested this method on 100 students (50 male and 50 female). The quality of life values the students ranged from 0.83 for the worst LUTS state to 0.96 for the best LUTS state. By comparison, the values for sexual dysfunction ranged from 0.74 (frequent problems) to 0.95 (seldom problems). The factor 'irritative' appeared to be rated as more severe than the factor 'obstructive'. These results are in line with those found in the literature. Our next step was to collect the ratings of the general public. Once the analysis of this data has been completed, we will have a final set of values specific for LUTS suggestive of BPO, which can then be used in economic evaluations within the Triumph project.

The Model

Statistical Analysis

The Triumph survey is a classical example of a naturalistic study that allows for a detailed estimation of the costs and effects in real practice. Using regression models, significant changes in patient status, such as change in therapy (to other medication or prostatic surgery), the development of serious complications related to BPO (e.g. AUR), change in Qol/I-PSS score, censoring and death will be examined. Separate analyses will be carried out for incident and prevalent cases. Using the information gathered from these analyses, we will build a model of the natural history of the disease.

It should be stressed that the statistical models may be country-specific or general. Where there is no evidence of statistically or clinically significant differences between countries, estimates of effects will be based on all available data. If such evidence exists, country-specific models will be used.

Cost-Effectiveness Survey

The cost-effectiveness survey will contain two components. One component will consist of a straightforward cost-effectiveness analysis of the various treatment modalities using the clinical effectiveness data gathered from the Triumph survey in combination with the average cost-estimates from the national costing databases. Given the follow-up period of the survey (1 year prospectively and about 3.5 years retrospectively), this survey will essentially present a snapshot, and hence a short-term, picture of the cost-effectiveness of current treatment regimes.

The second component will seek to provide a longer-term view and to examine the possible effects of altering the present treatment regimes (scenario analysis). This component will be based on a computer simulation model, using the country-specific demographic data, regression models and cost data. The computer model will simulate the progress of a large cohort of patients whose demographic characteristics are similar to those of each particular country. Each patient will be simulated individually and will be followed up for a number of years or until death. Initially, the patient will be randomly 'assigned' an initial I-PSS score and will then be 'assigned' to a treatment group and will subsequently 'progress' through the disease process, experiencing a change in his I-PSS score, undergoing therapy, including changes in therapy, possibly developing new serious complications related to BPO or new comorbidities, etc. All changes will be made according to the appropriate regression functions, or, where necessary, to estimates of longer-term effects of treatment etc derived from historical databases such as the GPRD or the IPCI databases. At each stage in a patient's progress, estimates of his I-PSS/QOL and associated costs of treatment of LUTS suggestive of BPO, complications and comorbidity will be made. At the end of follow-up, we have both a QOL and cost profile for each patient. These profiles will be used to calculate measures of treatment cost, effectiveness and cost-effectiveness.

Using these profiles, we can also examine the effect of implementing a number of treatment scenarios not currently implemented in Europe. For example, plant extracts are widely used in some European countries but are not used at all in others. One scenario might involve the removal of these plant extracts from all countries to examine their impact on cost-effectiveness. An alternative scenario might be to 'allow' its use in all European countries. Another scenario might be replacing watchful waiting (i.e. no medication but follow-up) with medical therapy. Another example is the choice of alpha-blocker within countries. For example, indoramin is widely used within the UK but is less widely used in other European countries. This raises the question as to whether the use of this alpha-blocker should be encouraged within other countries or discouraged within the UK.

Conclusions

Given the ageing of western populations, the cost burden associated with the treatment of LUTS suggestive of BPO will increase substantially over the next few decades; for example, Polder et al. [4] have estimated that the cost of treatment for BPH in the Netherlands will be more than double the present level by 2035. This burden will necessarily be borne by a decreasing proportion of the population. The Triumph project will allow us to examine the costs associated with LUTS suggestive of BPO and to measure the cost-effectiveness of the existing treatment regimes currently applied in Europe. These analyses, together with the scenario analyses, will provide greatly improved insight into the most cost-effective treatments for LUTS suggestive of BPO.

References

1 Welch, G, Kawachi I, Barry MJ, Giovannucci E, Colditz GA, Willett WC: Distinction between symptoms of voiding and filling in benign prostatic hyperplasia: Findings from the Health Professionals Follow-up Study. Urology 1998;51:422–427.

2 Drummond MF, O'Brien B, Stoddart GL, Torrance GW: Methods for the economic evaluation of health care programmes. Oxford, Oxford University Press, 1997.

3 Stolk EA, Busschbach JJV, Caffa M, Meuleman EJH, Rutten FFH: Cost utility analysis of sildenafil compared with papaverine-phentolamine injections. BMJ 2000;320:1165–1168.

4 Polder JJ, Meerding WJ, Koopmanschap MA, Bonneux L, van der Maas PJ: The cost of disease in the Netherlands (in Dutch). Institute of Medical Technology Assessment, 1994.

European Urology

Eur Urol 2001;39(suppl 3):42–47

Lower Urinary Tract Symptoms Suggestive of Benign Prostatic Obstruction – Triumph: The Role of General Practice Databases

John W. Logie[a] Gary M. Clifford[a] Richard D.T. Farmer[a]
Bianca P.W. Meesen[b]

[a]Department of Pharmacoepidemiology and Public Health, Postgraduate Medical School, University of Surrey, Guildford, UK; [b]Ismar Healthcare NV, Lier, Belgium

Key Words

Lower urinary tract symptoms · Benign prostatic obstruction · Long-term effectiveness · Triumph · Electronic patient record · Primary care · GRPD · IPCI · THALES

Abstract

The Triumph project aims to document the current management of lower urinary tract symptoms (LUTS) suggestive of benign prostatic hyperplasia (BPH) in general practice and to assess the effectiveness of the initial treatment options used. The first phase of the project will consider existing data sources in primary care. A patient's medical record will contain most, if not all, clinically relevant information, and databases combining the records from a network of computerised general practices can provide longitudinal data for complete populations, linking prescribing records to clinical information on disease progression and outcomes for individual patients. Database research can provide rapid information and offers the ability to conduct studies on a scale that would previously have been prohibited by both time and expense. Within the Triumph project, the THALES, General Practice Research Database (GPRD) and Integrated Primary Care Information (IPCI) databases are, or will be, used to examine the current management of LUTS/BPH in France, the UK and the Netherlands respectively. Preliminary results from the UK General Practice Research Database (GPRD) showed that LUTS/BPH incidence increased linearly from the ages of 45 to 85 years (r^2 = 0.992) and prevalence increased from 3.5% to 35% for men in their late 40s and 80s respectively. With treatment failure defined as a change to another medical therapy, catheterisation or prostatic surgery, and accounting for age and year variation, patients receiving the older α_1-blockers (indoramin and prazosin) appeared to fail significantly earlier than those receiving finasteride. There was no significant difference between finasteride and the newer α_1-blockers (tamsulosin, alfuzosin, terazosin and doxazosin). Patterns of changes between products from the THALES database in France were broadly similar to those seen in the UK.

Introduction

Lower urinary tract symptoms (LUTS) suggestive of benign prostatic hyperplasia (BPH) is a common condition among older men and its prevalence increases with age [1–5]. Traditionally, treatment has been by 'watchful waiting' (a period of regular follow-up but with no specific treatment), until the symptoms become severe enough to

KARGER

Fax + 41 61 306 12 34
E-Mail karger@karger.ch
www.karger.com

0302–2838/01/0399–0042$17.50/0

Accessible online at:
www.karger.com/journals/eur

Prof. R.D.T. Farmer
Department of Pharmacoepidemiology and Public Health
Postgraduate Medical School, University of Surrey, Stirling House
Stirling Road, Surrey Research Park, Guildford GU2 7DJ (UK)
Tel. +44 1483 302239, Fax +44 1483 300359, E-Mail r.farmer@surrey.ac.uk

require prostatic surgery. More recently, alternatives to surgical intervention have become available in the form of pharmacological therapies and, for many patients, these are now the first line treatment for the urinary symptoms suggestive of benign prostatic obstruction (BPO). Treatment options now include the 5α-reductase inhibitor finasteride, α_1-adrenoceptor antagonists (the α_1-blockers alfuzosin, doxazosin, indoramin, prazosin, tamsulosin and terazosin) and, in some countries, phytotherapy.

In the past, research programmes have provided insight into the prevalence of LUTS/BPH in the general community [1, 6, 7] and the predominantly short-term efficacy (effect on LUTS and urinary flow) of the main pharmacological treatment options in clinical trials [8]. Little information is available on the long-term efficacy or effectiveness of these treatments. Furthermore, it is increasingly realised that much of the available information comes from selected populations of patients presenting to secondary care urologists who are likely to be the more symptomatic patients. In clinical trials, the strict inclusion and exclusion criteria within the study protocols can also lead to uncertainty about the applicability of the results to community populations, particularly amongst patients with co-morbidity and co-medication. Moreover, because the patients within clinical trials are specially recruited, rather than drawn from a general population of men with LUTS, accurate calculations of incidence and prevalence rates may not be possible. The Triumph (TransEuropean Research Into the Use of Management Policies for LUTS suggestive of BPH in Primary Healthcare) project sets out to evaluate how lower urinary tract symptoms suggestive of benign prostatic obstruction are currently managed in general practice in Europe and to determine the long-term effectiveness of initial treatment options utilised by primary care physicians (PCPs) [9]. For each of the participating countries the Triumph program aims to assess: (1) the incidence and prevalence of LUTS (mainly described as BPH or urinary frequency by general practitioners (GPs)); (2) which treatment options are initially prescribed in primary care; (3) the proportion of patients that change to another treatment; (4) the proportion of patients in each initial treatment group hospitalised and/or catheterised because of acute urinary retention, and (5) the proportion of patients who develop other serious complications related to BPO such as urinary tract infections or renal dysfunction.

The first phase of the project will try to provide answers to these questions based on existing sources in primary care.

Existing Sources for Extracting Healthcare Management and Effectiveness Data

Information on drug prescribing, such as that collected by Intercontinental Medical Statistics (IMS), shows considerable differences within Europe in the medical management of LUTS. In all countries α_1-adrenoceptor antagonists (α_1-blockers) are the most frequently prescribed therapeutic class. Phytotherapy is used extensively in France, Germany and Spain, whereas finasteride is widely prescribed in Italy, Poland and the UK [10]. However, drug-prescribing data alone cannot give an insight into the overall management of LUTS, or information on the effectiveness of these drugs. For this, studies following treatment and the progression of symptoms in individuals over time are required. While these data can be collected by recruiting and following suitable patients, as in the prospective trials within Triumph, such studies are often expensive and require several years of data collection and follow-up before meaningful results can be produced. In some countries, longitudinal patients records are routinely collected in general practice. These records allow GP prescribing to be linked to clinical information on symptoms, diagnoses and outcomes for individual patients. Thus, from these records, the opportunity exists to examine the natural history of diseases and the long-term effectiveness of the drugs used in their treatment.

The Use of General Practice Records

A patient's medical record will contain most, if not all, clinically relevant information. To date, however, a major difficulty in using general practice records for medical research has been that most are only paper-based. Although the information within them can be retrieved by classical chart review, this process is costly in terms of time, effort and financial expense, and is unlikely to deliver the required data in the short-term. Increasingly, however, where the GP acts as the point of access of the healthcare system (as in the UK, the Netherlands and some Scandinavian countries), primary care providers are using computerised systems to generate prescriptions and for the administrative and financial management of their practices. In the UK, more than 90% of practices are currently computerised and about 8% are believed to be effectively paperless, i.e. using electronic patient records as the primary source of information [11]. In these circumstances, and if the data are recorded in standard formats, records from many practices can be combined to

Table 1. Examples of available GP information databases in Europe

France	THALES
	Euraxi
Italy	Friuli-Venezia Giulia (FVG)
The Netherlands	Continuous Morbidity Registration
	Registration Network Family Practices
	Integrated Primary Care Information (IPCI)
UK	General Practice Research Database (GPRD)
	MediPlus
	Doctors Independent Network (DIN)

produce central databases. If the data collection is managed and quality assured, the information from these sources can then be used for research purposes. In Europe, several databases are now available where the data are continuously or periodically updated from general practice (table 1). Most contain anonymised information on the patients' demographics, medical and medication history, diagnostic test results, secondary care referrals and all clinically relevant medical events and hospitalisations, entered in a standardised form. To date, these databases have been predominantly used for post-marketing surveillance to assess the association between specific adverse events and the use of certain drugs. However, there is an increasing tendency to use them for public health and pharmacoepidemiological research.

The Use of General Practice Databases

General practice databases provide longitudinal data for individual patients, linking prescribing records to clinical information on disease progression and outcomes. They are population based and therefore include representative patients of all ages. Unlike classical studies based on selected samples of patients, GP databases contain records of complete populations, irrespective of their medical status, and are thus able to provide the denominators required to calculate incidence and prevalence rates. Much of the value of database studies relies on this generalisability, and considerations of the composition of the patient base forms a central part of the data validation process. However, the database can only provide the prevalence of diagnosed disease in the population or describe the incidence of presentation. Many men with LUTS do not seek medical care and will remain undetected in database studies.

The quality of the databases relies on physicians entering all relevant patient information. Although the data should be quality assured, and validation studies have confirmed the standard of the largest European databases [12–15], the completeness of the medical records may be an issue in some cases. It is up to the GP whether or not he includes a specific outcome within a medical record. Negative observations are rarely recorded. In a review of patient records, Jick et al. found that 87% of diagnoses mentioned in consultants letters were associated with a concordant record on the general practice research database [12]. For many diagnoses recording exceeds 90%, particularly where diagnostic codes are supplemented with therapy records (i.e. insulin prescriptions for diabetic patients). For rare conditions recording may be close to 100% [15]. Thus, the data are likely to be of an appropriate quality for research use. These data are collected at the time of consultation for the management of the patient rather than to answer research questions. Thus, the records contain only information collected routinely in clinical practice and as with all observational data, the potential exists for bias and confounding. Treatment assignments are not randomised and outcomes are likely to be affected by a patient's symptom status at the onset of treatment. Information on symptom severity, such as the International Prostate Symptom Score (I-PSS), that might be collected in prospective studies will be incomplete or missing for many patients. The questions asked, and the results produced, must always be interpreted with caution in the knowledge of the limitation of the datasets. Nevertheless, once the research questions have been defined and translated into relevant database-specific searches, database research can provide desired information in a relatively short time and database research offers the ability to conduct studies on a scale that would previously have been prohibited by both time and expense. Where this is done, general practice databases can provide a powerful tool for epidemiological studies.

General Practice Databases within the Triumph Project

Within the Triumph project, the THALES database, General Practice Research Database (GPRD) and Integrated Primary Care Information database (IPCI) are, or will be, used to assess the current management of LUTS/BPH and the effectiveness of initial treatment options in France, the UK and the Netherlands, respectively.

THALES is a nation-wide computerised network of more than 600 representative GPs managing approximately 1 million patients in France (almost 2% of the total French population) [16]). The electronic patient records contain longitudinal information on patient characteristics, diagnoses and drug prescriptions. Importantly, this database does not contain data from secondary care such as medical events requiring hospitalisation or in-hospital interventions. Nevertheless, unlike IMS, which provides no information of prescribing to individual patients, the THALES database can provide data on the duration of treatment and changes between medical therapies. Initial analyses from the THALES database, show comparable utilisation patterns to those from IMS, suggesting that the GPs participating in this automated network will provide appropriate data for investigations into the management of LUTS in France.

The UK General Practice Research Database (GPRD) is Europe's largest computerised database of anonymised longitudinal patient records, currently covering a population of about 4.6 million people. It has been widely used for (pharmaco-)epidemiological and health service research [11, 17–23], and is currently owned and quality-controlled by the UK Medicines Control Agency (MCA) [24]. Practices have to undergo training in the use of the system and the quality of data has been high since 1992. Practices that fail to maintain the required standards are removed. Diagnoses are coded by a system developed for the VAMP Medical software (the OXMIS medical codes) which is loosely based on the International Classification of Diseases, 9th revision (ICD-9), or using Read codes, the coding system adopted by the UK Departments of Health for general practice [25]. Prescriptions are coded according to the Prescription Pricing Authority (PPA) codes. The geographical distribution of the practices participating in the GPRD is generally similar to that of the UK population, and comparisons of age and sex distributions with the national population census has shown them to be very similar [17].

The Integrated Primary Care Information (IPCI) database of the Erasmus University Medical School in Rotterdam is a GPRD-like database initiated in 1992 [26, 27]. There are about 6,500 GPs in the Netherlands with an average practice size of 2,400 patients [26]. In the Netherlands, the GP initially deals with about 90% of the patients' problems, the remaining 10% being referred to a specialist [26]. Although patients are free to change GP, most remain with the same practitioner. Currently, 150 GPs managing 485,000 patients (about 3% of the total Dutch population) are contributing to the semi-anonymous IPCI database. These practices are entirely computerised i.e. the practices are 'paperless' [26, 27], ensuring that the electronic patient records are as complete as possible. The files include information on patient characteristics, symptoms, prescriptions, indications for therapy, physical findings, laboratory test results, patient complaints, referral notes from consultation and hospital admissions, together with additional patient information such as smoking, alcohol consumption etc. Diagnoses and prescriptions are coded by the International Classification of Primary Care (ICPC) system and the Anatomical, Therapeutic and Chemical (ATC) coding system respectively [26]. So far, this database has predominantly been used to examine specific adverse events associated with particular drugs [28–30].

The Use of Database Studies within Triumph

In the Triumph project, the THALES database has been used to assess the incidence and prevalence of LUTS in France and to describe the initial treatment options used in primary care together with changes between these treatments. The GPRD will provide similar information for the UK and be used to examine secular trends in prescription for LUTS and the proportions of 'failures' for patients receiving each treatment. Within the analyses, a 'failure' is defined as a change in medical therapy, catheterisation or prostatic surgery. Each of these outcomes has been chosen to provide information on the efficacy and/or tolerability of the therapy a patient receives. The use of invasive treatments such as catheterisation or surgery, are normally determined by the severity of symptoms, and effective therapies should alleviate, or at least delay, the need for these procedures. The requirement for invasive therapy is likely, therefore, to be prompted by the failure of a treatment to manage a patient's symptoms adequately. Similarly, a patient is unlikely to change to an alternative drug therapy if their current medication is well tolerated and leading to a significant improvement in symptom severity. A change in therapy is taken to indicate dissatisfaction with the current treatment regime, either in terms of symptom progression or treatment tolerability. Currently, more than 110,000 men aged over 45 years with LUTS or a diagnosis of BPH have been identified from the GPRD, of which over 60,000 are incident cases being followed since their first presentation to primary care. Comparable analyses to those performed on the GPRD in the UK will be run on the Netherlands IPCI database.

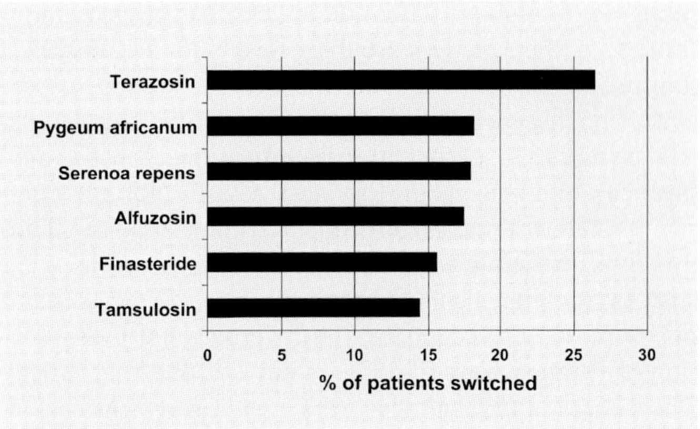

Fig. 1. Switches from the initial prescribed drug: results from the THALES database in France (1998; n = 1,738 incident cases) [16].

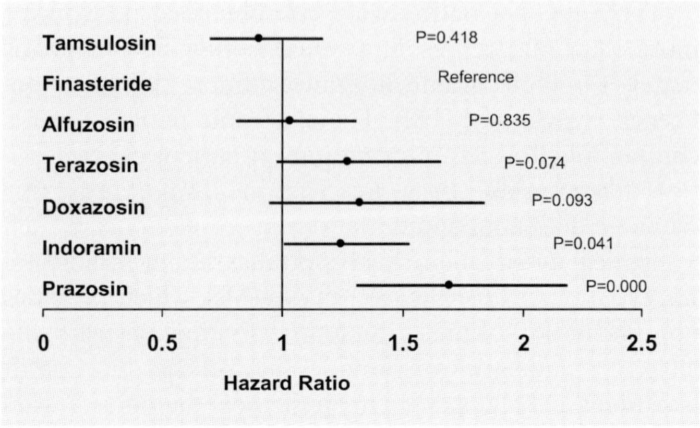

Fig. 3. Survival from first BPH/LUTS therapy to treatment failure (+CI_{95} adjusted for age and year): results from the GPRD in the UK [31].

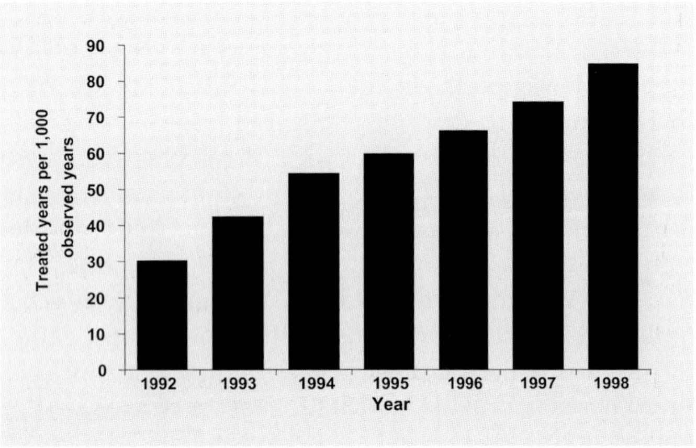

Fig. 2. Medically treated years per 1,000 LUTS/BPH years: results from the GPRD in the UK [31].

Preliminary Results

Preliminary analysis of the THALES database in France showed that approximately 50% of the men with LUTS received a prescription to relieve their symptoms. In 1998, around 50% of the prescriptions were for α-blockers, 35% for phytotherapy and 15% for finasteride. There was some evidence that the rate of changing to another medical therapy was lowest for tamsulosin and finasteride (fig. 1) [16].

A preliminary analysis of the GPRD assessed the incidence and prevalence of LUTS/BPH and the utilisation and effectiveness of initial therapy in 61,364 incident patients managed between 1992 and 1998 [31]. Incidence of LUTS increased linearly from the ages of 45 to 85 years (r^2 = 0.992), with prevalence increasing from 3.5% to 35% for men in their late 40s and 80s respectively. Prostatectomy rates increased linearly from the ages of 50 to 80 years (r^2 = 0.984). Between 1992 and 1998 there was a 3-fold increase in the proportion of time after first diagnosis of LUTS when patients were receiving medical therapy (fig. 2). This reflected the treatment of a greater proportion of symptomatic men, with these patients now appearing to receive therapy earlier in the disease progression than in the past. Patients are increasingly treated with newer medications (finasteride prior to 1996 and tamsulosin and alfuzosin since 1996) compared to older treatments (indoramin, prazosin). In addition, the interval between first diagnosis and prostatic surgery has increased progressively. Combining all products, patients receiving medical therapy came to prostatic surgery significantly later than those receiving no medication (Hazard ratio 0.76, 95% confidence interval 0.75–0.78). With a switch to other medical therapy, catheterisation or prostatic surgery as indications of product failure, and accounting for age and year variation, patients receiving the older α_1-blocker treatments (indoramin and prazosin) appeared to fail significantly earlier then those receiving finasteride (fig. 3). There was no significant difference between finasteride and the newer α_1-blocker medications (tamsulosin, alfuzosin, terazosin and doxazosin).

Similar analyses to those undertaken on the GPRD are currently being conducted on the IPCI database to assess whether these patterns are also evident in the Netherlands. In addition, updated analysis of both the GPRD and IPCI databases will be conducted in the coming years to see whether the observed trends are confirmed during longer follow-up.

Conclusions

General practice research databases can provide longitudinal data for complete populations, linking prescribing records to clinical information on disease progression and outcomes for individual populations. The data are observational, and the potential for bias and confounding exists. However, where appropriate research questions are asked and the results are interpreted with a knowledge of the limitations of the data, they offer the ability to conduct studies rapidly, and on a scale that would previously have been prohibited by both time and expense. They provide a valuable and powerful tool for epidemiological research.

References

1 Garraway WM, Collins GN, Lee RJ: High prevalence of benign prostatic hypertrophy in the community. Lancet 1991;338:469–471.
2 Bosch JLHR, Hop WJC, Kirkels WJ, Schröder FH: The International Prostate Symptom Score in a community-based sample of men between 55 and 74 years of age: Prevalence and correlation of symptoms with age, prostate volume, flow rate and residual urine volume. Br J Urol 1995;75:622–630.
3 Sagnier P-P, Macfarlane G, Richard F, Botto H, Teillac P, Boyle P: Results of an epidemiological survey using a modified American Urological Association symptom index for benign prostatic hyperplasia in France. J Urol 1994; 151:1266–1270.
4 Hunter DJW, Berra Unamuno A, Martin Gordo A: Prevalence of urinary symptoms and other urological conditions in Spanish men 50 years old or older. J Urol 1996;155:1965–1970.
5 Chicharro-Molero JA, Burgos-Rodriguez R, Sanchez-Cruz JJ, Del Rosal-Samaniego JM, Rodero-Carcia P, Rodriguez-Vallejo JM: Prevalence of benign prostatic hyperplasia in Spanish men 40 years old or older. J Urol 1998;159: 878–882.
6 Simpson RJ, Fisher W, Lee AJ, Russell EB, Garraway M: Benign prostatic hyperplasia in an unselected community-based population: A survey of urinary symptoms, bothersomeness and prostatic enlargement. BJU 1996;77:186–191.
7 Berry SJ, Coffey DS, Walsh PC, Ewing LL: The development of human benign prostatic hyperplasia with age. J Urol 1984;132:474–479.
8 Clifford GM, Farmer RDT: Medical therapy for benign prostatic hyperplasia: A review of the literature. Eur Urol 2000;38:2–19.
9 Chapple CR: Lower urinary tract symptoms suggestive of benign prostatic obstruction. Triumph: Design and implementation. Eur Urol 2001;39(suppl 3):31–36.
10 McNicholas T: Lower urinary tract symptoms suggestive of benign prostatic obstruction. What are the current practice patterns? Eur Urol 2001;39(suppl 3):26–30.
11 Lawrenson R, Williams T, Farmer R: Clinical information for research; the use of general practice databases. J Public Health Med 1999; 21:299–304.
12 Jick H, Jick SS, Derby LE: Validation of information recorded on general practitioner based computerised data resource in the United Kingdom [see comments]. BMJ 1991;302:766–768.
13 Hansell A, Hollowell J, Nichols T, McNiece R, Strachan D: Use of the General Practice Research Database (GPRD) for respiratory epidemiology: A comparison with the 4th Morbidity Survey in General Practice (MSGP4). Thorax 1999;54:413–419.
14 Nazareth I, King M, Haines A, Rangel L, Myers S: Accuracy of diagnosis of psychosis on general practice computer system. BMJ 1993; 307:32–34.
15 Van Staa T, Abenheim L: The quality of information recorded on general practitioner based computerised data resource in the United Kingdom. Pharmacoepidemiol Drug Safety 1994;3:15–21.
16 Vallancien G: How are lower urinary tract symptoms managed in real life practice? The French experience. Eur Urol 2000;38(suppl 1):54–59.
17 Garcia Rodriguez LA, Pérez-Gutthann S: Use of the UK General Practice Research Database for pharmacoepidemiology. Br J Clin Pharmacol 1998;45:419–425.
18 Farmer RDT, Williams TJ, Simpson EL, Nightingale AL: Effect of 1995 pill scare on rates of venous thromboembolism among women taking combined oral contraceptives: analysis of General Practice Research Database. BMJ 2000;321:477–479.
19 Farmer RDT, Lawrenson RA, Todd J-C, Williams TJ, MacRae KD, Tyrer F, Leydon GM: A comparison of the risks of venous thromboembolic disease in association with different combined oral contraceptives. Br J Clin Pharmacol 2000;49:580–590.
20 Soriano JB, Maier WC, Egger P, Visick G, Thakrar B, Sykes J, Pride NB: Recent trends in physician diagnosed COPD in women and men in the UK. Thorax 2000;55:789–794.
21 De Abajo FJ, Jick H, Derby L, Jick S, Schmitz S: Intracranial haemorrhage and use of selective serotonin reuptake inhibitors. Br J Clin Pharmacol 2000;50:43–47.
22 Meier CR, Schlienger RG, Kraenzlin ME, Schlegel B, Jick H: HMG-CoA reductase inhibitors and the risk of fractures. JAMA 2000;283: 3205–3210.
23 Hansell A, Hollowell J, Nichols T, McNiece R, Strachan D: Use of the General Practice Research Database (GPRD) for respiratory epidemiology: A comparison with the 4th Morbidity Survey in General Practice (MSGP4). Thorax 1999;54:413–419.
24 http://www.gprd.com
25 Saint Yves IF: The Read Clinical Classification. Hlth Bull Edinburgh 1992;50:422–427.
26 Vlug AE, Van der Lei J, Mosseveld BMTh, Van Wijk MAM, Van der Linden PD, Sturkenboom MCJM, Van Bemmel JH: Postmarketing surveillance based on electronic patient records: the IPCI project. Method Inform Med 1999;38: 339–344.
27 http://www.ipci.nl
28 Visser LE, Stricker BHC, Vlug AE, Van der Lei J: Coughing to ACE-inhibitors: a case-control study with automated general practice data. Eur J Clin Pharmacol 1996;49:439–444.
29 Van der Linden PD, van der Lei J, Vlug AE, Stricker BHCh: Skin reactions to antibacterial agents in general practice. J Clin Epidemiol 1998;51:703–708.
30 Van der Linden PD, Van der Lei J, Nab HW, Knol A, Stricker BHCh: Achilles tendinitis associated with fluoroquinolones. Br J Clin Pharmacol 1999;48:433–437.
31 Clifford GM, Logie J, Farmer RDT: How do symptoms indicative of BPH progress in real life practice? The UK experience. Eur Urol 2000;38(suppl 1):48–53.

Subject Index

European Urology

α_1-Adrenoceptor antagonists 20
Acute urinary retention 20
Benign prostatic hyperplasia 13
– – obstruction 20, 26, 31, 37, 42
BPH 6
BPO 6
Clinical decision making 13
Cost-effectiveness 6, 31, 37
Disease progression 20
Economic model 37
Electronic patient record 42
Evidence-based medicine 6
Finasteride 20
GRPD 42
Healthcare delivery 26
Health-economics 37
IPCI 42
Long-term 20, 31
– effectiveness 42
Lower urinary tract symptoms 26, 31, 37, 42
LUTS 6, 13
Medical therapy 26, 31
Practice guidelines 13
Primary care 26, 42
Progression to surgery 20
QALY 37
Rational management 6
Secondary care 26
Surgery 26
THALES 42
Treatment failure 31
Triumph 31, 42

KARGER
Fax + 41 61 306 12 34
E-Mail karger@karger.ch
www.karger.com

Accessible online at:
www.karger.com/journals/eur

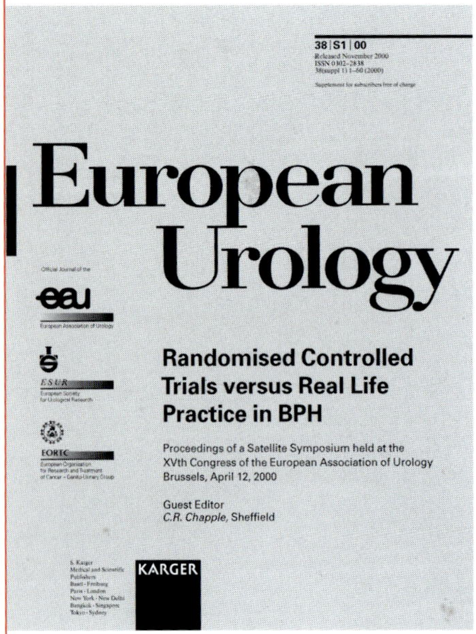
38 | S1 | 00
Released November 2000
ISSN 0302–2838
38(suppl 1) 1–60 (2000)

European Urology

Official Journal of the
eau
European Association of Urology
ESUR
European Society for Urological Research
EORTC
European Organization for Research and Treatment of Cancer – Genito-Urinary Group

Randomised Controlled Trials versus Real Life Practice in BPH

Proceedings of a Satellite Symposium held at the XVth Congress of the European Association of Urology Brussels, April 12, 2000

Guest Editor
C.R. Chapple, Sheffield

S. Karger
Medical and Scientific Publishers
Basel · Freiburg
Paris · London
New York · New Delhi
Bangkok · Singapore
Tokyo · Sydney

KARGER

Randomised Controlled Trials versus Real Life Practice in BPH

Guest Editor
C.R. Chapple

Urology

Contents

Introduction and Concluding Remarks: ***Chapple, C.R.***

Invasive and Minimally Invasive Treatment Modalities for Lower Urinary Tract Symptoms: What Are the Relevant Differences in Randomised Controlled Trials? ***Tubaro, A.; Vicentini, C.; Renzetti, R.; Miano, L.***

Medical Treatment Modalities for Lower Urinary Tract Symptoms: What Are the Relevant Differences in Randomised Controlled Trials? ***Zimmern, P.***

α_1-Blocker Therapy for Lower Urinary Tract Symptoms Suggestive of Benign Prostatic Obstruction: What Are the Relevant Differences in Randomised Controlled Trials? ***De Mey, C.***

Treatment Satisfaction of Patients with Lower Urinary Tract Symptoms: Randomised Controlled Trials vs. Real Life Practice: ***Michel, M.C.; Goepel, M.***

How Do Symptoms Indicative of BPH Progress in Real Life Practice? The UK Experience: ***Clifford, G.M.; Logie, J.; Farmer, R.D.T.***

How Are Lower Urinary Tract Symptoms Managed in Real Life Practice? The French Experience: ***Vallancien, G.***

Subject Index

KI 00693

www.karger.com/journals/eur

European Urology
Editor: Schulman, C.C. (Brussels)
ISSN 0302–2838
Supplement issue: Vol. 38, Suppl. 1 (2000)
Included in subscription

Randomised Controlled Trials versus Real Life Practice in BPH
Proceedings of a Satellite Symposium held at the XVth Congress of the European Association of Urology
Editor: Chapple, C.R. (Sheffield)
60 p., 21 fig., 6 tab., soft cover, 2000
CHF 29.– / DEM 38.– / USD 25.25
Prices subject to change
DEM price for Germany, USD price for USA only
ISBN 3–8055–7181–X

KARGER

Order Form

Please send: ____ copy/ies

Postage and handling free with prepayment

Payment:
☐ Check enclosed ☐ Please bill me

Please charge to my credit card
☐ American Express ☐ Diners ☐ Eurocard
☐ MasterCard ☐ Visa

Card No.: ____________________

Exp. date: ____________________

☐ Please send a free sample copy of the journal **European Urology**

Orders may be placed with any bookshop, subscription agency, directly with the publisher or through a Karger distributor.

Fax: +41 61 306 12 34
S. Karger AG, P.O. Box, CH–4009 Basel (Switzerland)
E-Mail karger@karger.ch, **www.karger.com**

Name/Address: ____________________

Date: ____________________

Signature: ____________________